EMPOWERING WOMEN THROUGH CBT: STRATEGIES FOR OVERCOMING ANXIETY, DEPRESSION, AND LOW SELF-ESTEEM

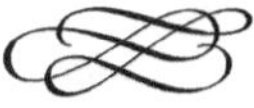

ALICE JENNIFER

CONTENTS

UNDERSTANDING CBT: AN INTRODUCTION TO COGNITIVE BEHAVIOR THERAPY FOR WOMEN

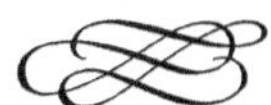

elcome to the world of Cognitive Behavior Therapy (CBT), a powerful tool that has helped countless women overcome mental health challenges and lead more fulfilling lives. In this chapter, we'll dive into the core principles of CBT and explore how they relate specifically to women's mental health. We'll also take a closer look at the benefits of CBT for managing anxiety, depression, and low self-esteem, three common issues that many women face.

So, what exactly is CBT? At its core, CBT is a form of psychotherapy that focuses on the relationship between our thoughts, feelings, and behaviors. The main idea behind CBT is that our thoughts have a significant impact on how we feel and behave. When we experience negative or distorted thoughts, it can lead to emotional distress and unhelpful behaviors. CBT aims to help individuals identify and change these negative thought patterns, leading to improved mental health and well-being.

One of the key principles of CBT is that our thoughts are not always accurate reflections of reality. Sometimes, our minds can play tricks on us, causing us to interpret situations in a negative or distorted way. For example, let's say you're preparing for a job interview. You might find yourself thinking, "I'm not good enough for this job. I'll probably mess up the interview and embarrass myself." These thoughts are not based on facts but rather on your own self-doubts and fears. CBT helps you recognize these negative thought patterns and challenges them with evidence and more balanced perspectives.

So, why is this particularly important for women? Research has shown that women are more likely than men to experience certain mental health issues, such as anxiety and depression. There are many factors that contribute to this gender disparity, including biological differences, societal pressures, and gender roles. Women often face unique stressors, such as balancing work and family responsibilities, dealing with body image issues, and navigating societal expectations. These stressors can take a toll on mental health and lead to negative thought patterns.

For example, let's consider the issue of body image. From a young age, girls are bombarded with messages about what the "ideal" female body should look like. They see images of thin, photoshopped models in magazines and on social media, and they may feel pressure to conform to these unrealistic standards. As a result, many women develop negative thoughts about their own bodies, such as "I'm too fat" or "I'm not pretty enough." These thoughts can lead to low self-esteem, anxiety, and even eating disorders.

CBT can be a powerful tool for helping women challenge these negative thoughts about their bodies. A CBT therapist might ask a client to examine the evidence for and against their negative body image thoughts. For example, a client might say, "I'm too fat." The therapist would then ask, "What evidence do you have for that thought? Have you ever known anyone that thought you were over-weight?" The client might realize that their thought is based on their own self-perception rather than reality. The therapist could then help the client develop more balanced and realistic thoughts, such as "My body is unique and deserves love and respect."

Another common issue that women face is imposter syndrome, which is the feeling of being a fraud or not being good enough, despite evidence of success. This can be particularly prevalent in the workplace, where women may feel pressure to prove themselves in male-dominated fields. A woman might think, "I only got this promotion because of luck. I don't really deserve it." CBT can help women challenge these thoughts and recognize their own strengths and accomplishments.

CBT can also be beneficial for women who struggle with anxiety. Anxiety is characterized by excessive worry and fear, often about future events or potential dangers. Women are more likely than men to experience anxiety disorders, such as generalized anxiety disorder, panic disorder, and social anxiety disorder. CBT can help women learn to manage their anxiety by identifying and challenging their anxious thoughts.

Here's an example: A woman with social anxiety disorder might have the thought, "Everyone at this party is judging me. They think I'm awkward and boring." This thought can lead to feelings of intense anxiety and even avoidance of social situations. In CBT, the therapist would help the woman examine the evidence for and against this thought. The therapist might ask, "How do you know that everyone is judging you negatively? Are there any other possible explanations for their behavior?" The woman might realize that her anxiety is causing her to interpret neutral or even positive social cues as negative. With practice, she can learn to challenge these anxious thoughts and approach social situations with more confidence.

Depression is another common mental health issue that affects women at higher rates than men. Depression is characterized by persistent feelings of sadness, hopelessness, and low energy. Women may experience depression due to a variety of factors, including hormonal changes, life stressors, and past trauma. CBT can be an effective treatment for depression in women, helping them to identify and change negative thought patterns.

One common negative thought pattern in depression is overgeneralization, which is the tendency to view a single negative event as a never-ending pattern of defeat. For example, a woman who experiences a breakup might think, "I'll never find love again. I'm destined to be alone forever." CBT would help this woman recognize that this thought is an overgeneralization and not based on reality. The therapist might encourage the woman to look for evidence that challenges this thought, such as past experiences of resilience and strength.

Another benefit of CBT for women is that it can help improve self-esteem. Low self-esteem is a common issue among women, often rooted in negative experiences and messages received throughout life. A woman with low self-esteem might have thoughts like "I'm not good enough" or "I don't deserve happiness." CBT can help women challenge these negative self-beliefs and develop a more positive and compassionate view of themselves.

One technique that CBT therapists use to help improve self-esteem is positive self-talk. This involves identifying negative self-talk (such as "I'm a failure") and replacing it with more positive and realistic statements (such as "I'm doing my best and learning from my mistakes"). The therapist might also encourage the woman to engage in activities that promote self-care and self-compassion, such as taking a relaxing bath or practicing mindfulness.

CBT can also be beneficial for women who have experienced trauma, such as sexual assault or domestic violence. Trauma can have a profound impact on mental health, leading to symptoms such as flashbacks, nightmares, and avoidance of triggering situations. CBT can help women process their traumatic experiences and develop coping strategies for managing symptoms.

One specific type of CBT that is often used for trauma is cognitive processing therapy (CPT). CPT helps individuals challenge and modify unhelpful beliefs related to the trauma, such as self-blame or mistrust of others. The therapist might ask the client to write a detailed account of the traumatic event and then help them identify and challenge any distorted thoughts or beliefs related to the event. Through this process, the client can begin to develop a more balanced and healthy perspective on the trauma.

It's important to note that CBT is not a one-size-fits-all approach to mental health treatment. While it can be highly effective for many women, it may not be the best fit for everyone. Some women may prefer other types of therapy, such as mindfulness-based therapies or interpersonal therapy. It's important for women to work with a qualified mental health professional to determine the best treatment approach for their individual needs.

In conclusion, CBT is a powerful tool that can help women overcome a wide range of mental health challenges, including anxiety, depression, low self-esteem, and trauma. By identifying and challenging negative thought patterns, women can develop more balanced and realistic perspectives on themselves and the world around them. CBT can also help women build resilience and coping skills that can serve them throughout their lives. If you're a woman struggling with mental health issues, consider seeking out a qualified CBT therapist to help you on your journey towards healing and empowerment.

IDENTIFYING NEGATIVE THOUGHT PATTERNS AND THEIR IMPACT ON WOMEN'S MENTAL HEALTH

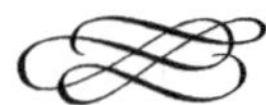

In the previous chapter, we explored the basics of Cognitive Behavior Therapy (CBT) and how it can be a valuable tool for improving women's mental health. Now, let's dive deeper into one of the key components of CBT: identifying negative thought patterns and understanding how they contribute to anxiety, depression, and low self-esteem.

Negative thought patterns are habitual ways of thinking that are often biased, inaccurate, or exaggerated. These thoughts can be so automatic and ingrained that we may not even realize we're having them. However, they can have a profound impact on our emotions and behaviors, leading to mental health challenges like anxiety and depression.

Women, in particular, are prone to certain types of negative thought patterns. One common pattern is self-criticism. Women often hold themselves to impossibly high standards and berate themselves for even minor mistakes or imperfections. For example, a woman might think, "I'm so stupid for forgetting that appointment. I can't do anything right." This type of self-talk is harmful because it chips away at self-esteem and reinforces feelings of inadequacy.

Another negative thought pattern that is common among women

is perfectionism. Perfectionism is the belief that anything less than perfect is unacceptable. Women may feel pressure to excel in all areas of life, from work to relationships to appearance. They may set unrealistic goals for themselves and then feel like failures when they inevitably fall short. For example, a woman might think, "If I don't get a promotion this year, it means I'm not good enough at my job." This type of all-or-nothing thinking can lead to chronic stress and burnout.

So why are women particularly prone to these negative thought patterns? There are a few key factors at play. One is societal pressure. From a young age, girls are bombarded with messages about how they should look, behave, and achieve. They may internalize the idea that their worth is tied to their appearance, their relationship status, or their professional success. This can create a constant sense of pressure to measure up to an impossible standard.

Another factor is the way that women are socialized to prioritize the needs of others over their own. Women are often expected to be caretakers and nurturers, putting the needs of their family, friends, and colleagues ahead of their own. This can lead to a sense of self-sacrifice and a belief that one's own needs and desires are less important. A woman might think, "I can't take a day off work to rest, even though I'm exhausted. My team needs me too much." This type of thinking can lead to burnout and a lack of self-care.

Negative thought patterns can also be reinforced by past experiences and traumas. Women who have experienced abuse, discrimination, or other forms of trauma may develop negative beliefs about themselves and the world around them. For example, a woman who was bullied as a child for her appearance might develop the belief that she is ugly and unlovable. These negative beliefs can be difficult to shake, even years later.

So how do these negative thought patterns contribute to anxiety, depression, and low self-esteem? Let's take a closer look.

Anxiety is characterized by excessive worry and fear about future events. Women who engage in negative thought patterns may be more prone to anxiety because they are constantly anticipating the worst-case scenario. For example, a woman who is self-critical might worry that she will make a mistake at work and get fired. A woman who is a perfectionist might worry that she will never be able to meet her own high standards. These types of thoughts can create a constant sense of unease and tension.

Depression, on the other hand, is characterized by persistent feelings of sadness, hopelessness, and worthlessness. Negative thought patterns can contribute to depression by reinforcing feelings of inadequacy and despair. For example, a woman who is self-critical might believe that she is a failure and that nothing she does will ever be good enough. A woman who has experienced trauma might believe that she is permanently damaged and that happiness is out of reach. These types of thoughts can create a downward spiral of negative emotions.

Low self-esteem is another common issue that can be exacerbated by negative thought patterns. Self-esteem refers to the way we feel about ourselves and our sense of self-worth. Women who engage in self-criticism or perfectionism may have chronically low self-esteem because they are constantly finding fault with themselves. They may feel like they are never good enough, no matter how much they achieve. This can lead to a lack of confidence and a fear of taking risks or trying new things.

So what can women do to break free from these negative thought patterns? The first step is to become aware of them. Many negative thoughts are so automatic that we don't even realize we're having them. One way to increase awareness is to keep a thought diary. This involves writing down negative thoughts as they occur, along with the situation that triggered them and the emotions they provoked. For example:

Situation: I made a mistake at work and my boss pointed it out in front of my colleagues. Negative thought: I'm such an idiot. I can't do anything right. Emotion: Shame, embarrassment, anxiety

By writing down negative thoughts, women can start to recognize patterns and triggers. They may notice that certain situations, like public speaking or social events, consistently provoke negative self-talk. They may also notice that certain types of thoughts, like self-criticism or catastrophizing (assuming the worst will happen), are particularly common.

Once women have identified their negative thought patterns, they can start to challenge them. This involves examining the evidence for and against the thought and considering alternative perspectives. For example, a woman who thinks "I'm such an idiot" after making a mistake at work might ask herself:

• What evidence do I have that I'm an idiot? Have I made mistakes before and still been successful overall?

• What would I say to a friend who made a similar mistake? Would I be as hard on them as I am on myself?

• Are there any other possible explanations for my mistake, like being tired or stressed?

By challenging negative thoughts, women can start to develop a more balanced and realistic perspective. They may realize that their thoughts are overly harsh or not based on facts. They may also develop more self-compassion and learn to treat themselves with kindness and understanding.

Another strategy for overcoming negative thought patterns is to practice positive self-talk. This involves intentionally replacing negative thoughts with more positive and empowering ones. For example, instead of thinking "I'm a failure," a woman might tell herself "I'm doing my best and learning from my mistakes." Instead of thinking "I'll never be good enough," she might tell herself "I am worthy and deserving of love and respect."

Positive self-talk can feel awkward or unnatural at first, especially for women who are used to being self-critical. It can help to start small, with simple affirmations like "I am strong" or "I am capable." Over time, women can build up to more specific and personal affirmations, like "I am a talented writer" or "I am a caring and supportive friend."

It's also important for women to practice self-care and prioritize their own needs and well-being. This can involve setting boundaries, saying no to unreasonable requests, and making time for activities that bring joy and relaxation. For example, a woman who is feeling overwhelmed with work and family responsibilities might schedule a weekly yoga class or coffee date with a friend. These activities can help reduce stress and promote a sense of balance and well-being.

Finally, it's important for women to seek support when needed. Negative thought patterns can be stubborn and difficult to change on one's own. Working with a therapist who specializes in CBT can be incredibly helpful for identifying and challenging negative thoughts. Support groups can also be a valuable resource, providing a safe space to share experiences and learn from others who have struggled with similar issues.

In conclusion, negative thought patterns are a common challenge for women and can contribute to anxiety, depression, and low self-esteem. By becoming aware of these patterns, challenging them with evidence and alternative perspectives, practicing positive self-talk, prioritizing self-care, and seeking support when needed, women can break free from the cycle of negative thinking and develop a more positive and empowered mindset. Remember, change takes time and practice, but every small step towards more balanced and realistic thinking is a step towards improved mental health and well-being.

CHALLENGING AND REFRAMING NEGATIVE THOUGHTS: CBT TECHNIQUES FOR WOMEN

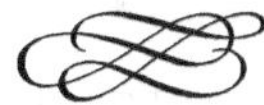

In the previous chapter, we explored how negative thought patterns can contribute to anxiety, depression, and low self-esteem in women. These thought patterns can be so automatic and ingrained that they feel like absolute truths, even when they are based on biased or inaccurate perceptions. The good news is that Cognitive Behavior Therapy (CBT) offers practical techniques for identifying, challenging, and reframing negative thoughts. In this chapter, we'll dive into these techniques and explore how they can help women develop a more positive and resilient mindset.

The first step in challenging negative thoughts is to become aware of them. Many women have negative self-talk that is so habitual that they don't even realize they're doing it. They may have thoughts like "I'm not good enough," "I'll never succeed," or "I'm a failure" running through their minds on a constant loop. These thoughts can be triggered by external events, like a criticism from a boss or a fight with a partner, or they may seem to come out of nowhere.

One way to increase awareness of negative thoughts is to practice mindfulness. Mindfulness involves paying attention to one's thoughts, feelings, and sensations in the present moment, without judgment. When a negative thought arises, a woman practicing mindfulness might notice it, acknowledge it, and then let it pass without getting caught up in it. For example, she might think, "I notice I'm having the thought that I'm not good enough. That's just a thought, not a fact."

Another way to increase awareness of negative thoughts is to keep a thought diary. This involves writing down negative thoughts as they occur, along with the situation that triggered them and the emotions they provoked. For example:

Situation: I got feedback on my work project and my supervisor pointed out some areas for improvement. Negative thought: I'm a terrible employee. I can't do anything right. Emotion: Shame, anxiety, frustration

By writing down negative thoughts, women can start to notice patterns and triggers. They may realize that they are more prone to negative self-talk in certain situations, like when they are stressed or tired. They may also notice that certain types of thoughts, like all-or-nothing thinking or catastrophizing, are particularly common.

Once women have identified their negative thoughts, they can start to challenge them. One common CBT technique for challenging negative thoughts is called "cognitive restructuring." This involves examining the evidence for and against the thought and considering alternative perspectives.

For example, let's say a woman has the thought "I'm a terrible mother." She might challenge this thought by asking herself:

• What evidence do I have that I'm a terrible mother? Have I made mistakes or had moments of frustration? Sure. But does that mean I'm a terrible mother overall?

• What evidence do I have that I'm a good mother? Do I love my children and try my best to meet their needs? Do I have moments of joy and connection with them?

• Are there any other possible explanations for my perceived failings as a mother? Am I comparing myself to an unrealistic standard or expecting perfection from myself?

By examining the evidence for and against the negative thought, the woman may realize that her self-assessment is overly harsh and not based on reality. She may develop a more balanced perspective, such as "I'm a loving and imperfect mother, just like everyone else."

Another CBT technique for challenging negative thoughts is called "reframing." This involves looking at a situation from a different perspective or finding a silver lining. For example, a woman who is upset about a recent breakup might reframe her thinking from "I'll never find love again" to "This is an opportunity for me to focus on my own personal growth and happiness."

Reframing can be particularly helpful for women who tend to catastrophize or assume the worst will happen. For example, a woman who is worried about a upcoming job interview might have the thought "I'm going to embarrass myself and ruin my chances of getting hired." She could reframe this thought by telling herself, "This is an opportunity for me to showcase my skills and experience. Even if I don't get the job, it will be a valuable learning experience."

It's important to note that reframing doesn't mean ignoring or minimizing negative emotions. It's okay to feel sad, anxious, or angry in response to difficult situations. However, reframing can help prevent negative emotions from spiraling out of control or leading to unhelpful behaviors.

In addition to cognitive restructuring and reframing, there are many other CBT techniques that can help women challenge negative thoughts. One is called "behavioral activation," which involves scheduling enjoyable or meaningful activities to boost mood and counteract negative thinking. For example, a woman who is feeling down about her job might schedule a weekly hike with friends or volunteer at a local animal shelter. These activities can provide a sense of accomplishment and social connection, which can help combat negative self-talk.

Another technique is called "exposure therapy," which involves gradually confronting feared situations or objects to reduce anxiety and build confidence. For example, a woman who is afraid of public speaking might start by practicing speeches in front of a mirror, then in front of a trusted friend, and eventually in front of a larger group. By facing her fear in a controlled and gradual way, she can learn that she is capable of handling the situation and that her negative predictions (e.g., "I will faint or vomit during my speech") are unlikely to come true.

A third technique is called "problem-solving," which involves breaking down a challenging situation into smaller, more manageable steps. For example, a woman who is overwhelmed by a large work project might break it down into smaller tasks and create a timeline for completing each one. This can help her feel more in control and less prone to negative self-talk like "I can't handle this" or "I'm going to fail."

It's important for women to find the CBT techniques that work best for them and to practice them regularly. Like any skill, challenging negative thoughts takes time and effort to master. Women may find it helpful to work with a therapist who specializes in CBT, as they can provide guidance and support in identifying and changing negative thought patterns.

It's also important for women to be patient and compassionate with themselves as they work on challenging negative thoughts. It's normal to have setbacks or moments of self-doubt, especially when dealing with long-standing thought patterns. The key is to keep practicing and to celebrate small victories along the way.

One way to stay motivated is to focus on the benefits of challenging negative thoughts. Women who are able to reframe their thinking and develop a more positive outlook may experience a range of benefits, including:

- Increased self-esteem and self-confidence
- Reduced symptoms of anxiety and depression
- Improved relationships and communication skills
- Greater resilience in the face of stress and adversity
- Increased motivation and productivity
- Enhanced overall well-being and life satisfaction

By reminding themselves of these benefits, women can stay committed to the process of challenging negative thoughts, even when it feels difficult or uncomfortable.

It's also important for women to surround themselves with

supportive people who can provide encouragement and perspective. This might include friends, family members, or a therapist. Having a strong support system can make it easier to challenge negative thoughts and maintain a positive outlook.

Finally, women may find it helpful to practice self-care and stress management techniques in addition to challenging negative thoughts. This might include activities like exercise, meditation, journaling, or creative hobbies. By taking care of their physical and emotional needs, women can build resilience and reduce their vulnerability to negative thinking.

In conclusion, challenging and reframing negative thoughts is a crucial skill for women who want to improve their mental health and well-being. CBT offers a range of practical techniques for identifying, examining, and changing negative thought patterns, including cognitive restructuring, reframing, behavioral activation, exposure therapy, and problem-solving. By practicing these techniques regularly and seeking support when needed, women can develop a more positive and resilient mindset that enables them to thrive in all areas of life. Remember, change takes time and effort, but every small step towards more balanced and realistic thinking is a step towards greater happiness and fulfillment.

BUILDING SELF-ESTEEM AND SELF-COMPASSION THROUGH CBT

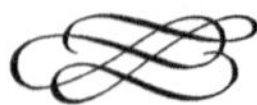

In the previous chapters, we explored the basics of Cognitive Behavior Therapy (CBT) and how it can be used to identify and challenge negative thought patterns that contribute to anxiety, depression, and low self-esteem in women. Now, let's dive deeper into two crucial components of mental health and well-being: self-esteem and self-compassion.

Self-esteem refers to the way we view and value ourselves. It encompasses our beliefs about our worth, competence, and lovability. Women with healthy self-esteem tend to have a positive and realistic view of themselves, their abilities, and their potential. They are able to acknowledge their strengths and weaknesses, and they treat themselves with kindness and respect.

On the other hand, women with low self-esteem may have a distorted and overly critical view of themselves. They may focus on their flaws and failures, and dismiss their positive qualities and accomplishments. They may engage in negative self-talk, such as "I'm not good enough," "I'm a failure," or "I don't deserve happiness." Low self-esteem can lead to a range of mental health challenges, including anxiety, depression, and relationship problems.

Self-compassion, a related concept, refers to the ability to treat oneself with kindness, care, and understanding, particularly in the face of difficult emotions or experiences. It involves recognizing that suffering and imperfection are part of the shared human experience, and that we all deserve compassion and support. Women who practice self-compassion are able to comfort and soothe themselves during tough times, rather than engaging in self-criticism or blame.

Research has shown that self-compassion is strongly linked to mental health and well-being. Women who are more self-compassionate tend to have lower levels of anxiety and depression, higher levels of happiness and life satisfaction, and more fulfilling relationships. They are also more resilient in the face of stress and adversity, and more likely to engage in healthy behaviors like exercise and self-care.

Unfortunately, many women struggle with low self-esteem and a lack of self-compassion. This can be due to a variety of factors, including societal pressures, past experiences of trauma or abuse, and internalized messages about gender roles and expectations. Women may feel pressure to be perfect, to prioritize others' needs over their own, and to base their worth on their appearance, relationships, or achievements.

The good news is that CBT offers a range of techniques for building self-esteem and self-compassion. These techniques can help women develop a more positive and accepting relationship with themselves, even in the face of challenges and setbacks.

One key technique for building self-esteem is cognitive restructuring, which involves identifying and challenging negative beliefs about oneself. For example, a woman with low self-esteem might have the belief "I'm not smart enough to succeed in my career." Through cognitive restructuring, she could examine the evidence for and against this belief, and consider alternative perspectives.

She might ask herself questions like:

• What evidence do I have that I'm not smart enough? Have I had successes in my career that suggest otherwise?

• Are there any other factors that contribute to career success besides intelligence, such as hard work, persistence, and networking?

• What would I say to a friend who had this same belief about themselves? Would I be as harsh and critical, or would I offer encouragement and support?

By challenging the negative belief and considering more balanced and realistic perspectives, the woman can start to build a more positive view of herself and her abilities.

Another CBT technique for building self-esteem is positive self-talk. This involves intentionally replacing negative self-talk with more affirming and compassionate messages. For example, instead of telling herself "I'm a failure," a woman could practice saying "I'm doing my best and learning from my mistakes."

Positive self-talk can feel awkward or unnatural at first, especially for women who are used to being self-critical. It can help to start with small, believable statements and gradually work up to more challenging ones. For example, a woman who struggles with body image might start by telling herself "My body allows me to do the things I love, like hiking and dancing," before moving on to more global statements like "I am beautiful and worthy of love and respect."

It's important to practice positive self-talk regularly, even when it feels difficult or uncomfortable. Over time, it can help reprogram the brain to focus on positive aspects of oneself and build a more resilient sense of self-worth.

Another key technique for building self-compassion is mindfulness. Mindfulness involves bringing one's attention to the present moment with openness, curiosity, and non-judgment. When difficult emotions or experiences arise, mindfulness can help women respond with kindness and understanding, rather than self-criticism or avoidance.

For example, let's say a woman experiences a painful rejection from a romantic partner. A self-critical response might be to blame herself and engage in negative self-talk, such as "I'm unlovable" or "I'll never find happiness." A mindful and self-compassionate response, on the other hand, might sound something like this:

"This feeling of rejection is so painful. It's natural to feel sad and hurt when a relationship ends. I'm not alone in experiencing this kind of pain – it's a normal part of the human experience. I'm going to be extra kind and gentle with myself as I navigate this difficult time."

By acknowledging the pain of the experience without judgment, and offering herself compassion and support, the woman can start to heal and move forward in a healthy way.

Another way to practice self-compassion is through loving-kindness meditation. This involves silently repeating phrases of goodwill and compassion towards oneself and others, such as "May I be happy, may I be healthy, may I be at peace." Research has shown that regular loving-kindness meditation can increase feelings of self-compassion, as well as compassion towards others.

In addition to these CBT techniques, there are many other ways that women can build self-esteem and self-compassion in their daily lives. One is to practice gratitude by regularly acknowledging the good things in one's life, such as supportive relationships, personal strengths, and moments of joy and beauty. Keeping a gratitude journal or sharing appreciations with loved ones can help cultivate a more positive and appreciative mindset.

Another way to build self-esteem and self-compassion is to engage in activities that bring a sense of mastery, purpose, or flow. This might include hobbies like painting, gardening, or playing an instrument, or pursuing meaningful goals like volunteering or learning a new skill. By regularly engaging in activities that challenge and fulfill us, we can build a sense of competence and worth that is not dependent on external validation.

It's also important for women to practice self-care and set healthy boundaries in their relationships and responsibilities. This might involve saying no to unreasonable requests, carving out time for rest and relaxation, or seeking support from a therapist or trusted friend. By prioritizing their own needs and well-being, women can send a powerful message to themselves that they are valuable and deserving of care and respect.

Of course, building self-esteem and self-compassion is not always easy, and it's normal to experience setbacks and challenges along the way. It's important for women to be patient and persistent in their efforts, and to seek support when needed.

One helpful resource for women seeking to build self-esteem and self-compassion is the work of Dr. Kristin Neff, a leading researcher in the field of self-compassion. Dr. Neff has developed a range of resources and exercises for cultivating self-compassion, including guided meditations, self-compassion breaks, and a self-compassion scale that can help women assess their current levels of self-kindness and mindfulness.

Another resource is the book "The Gifts of Imperfection" by Dr. Brené Brown, which explores the importance of cultivating self-compassion, authenticity, and vulnerability in order to live a whole-hearted and fulfilling life. Dr. Brown's work emphasizes the idea that our imperfections and struggles are not shameful or unlovable, but rather a natural and valuable part of the human experience.

Ultimately, building self-esteem and self-compassion is a lifelong journey that requires ongoing commitment and practice. By using CBT techniques like cognitive restructuring, positive self-talk, mindfulness, and loving-kindness meditation, and by seeking out supportive resources and relationships, women can gradually cultivate a more loving and accepting relationship with themselves.

The benefits of this work are profound and far-reaching. Women with healthy self-esteem and self-compassion are more likely to have fulfilling relationships, pursue their goals and dreams with confidence, and bounce back from setbacks and challenges with resilience and grace. They are also more likely to treat others with kindness and empathy, creating a ripple effect of positivity and connection in their families, workplaces, and communities.

In a world that often sends women messages of inadequacy and self-doubt, the cultivation of self-esteem and self-compassion is a radical and transformative act. It is a way of claiming our inherent worth and dignity, and of treating ourselves with the same love and respect that we so freely give to others.

As we conclude this chapter on building self-esteem and self-compassion through CBT, I invite you to reflect on your own relationship with yourself. What are the negative beliefs or self-talk patterns that you would like to challenge and reframe? What are the moments of joy, strengths, and accomplishments that you can celebrate and appreciate? What are the ways that you can practice self-kindness and self-care, even in the midst of life's challenges and imperfections?

Remember, you are worthy of love, respect, and compassion, simply by virtue of being human. By committing to the ongoing work of building self-esteem and self-compassion, you are not only transforming your own life, but also contributing to a world that is more loving, accepting, and kind. May you find the courage and support you need to take those first steps, and to keep going even when the path is difficult. You are worth it.

MANAGING ANXIETY WITH CBT: STRATEGIES FOR WOMEN

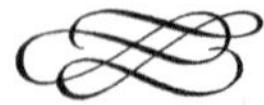

Anxiety is a common and often debilitating mental health challenge that affects millions of women worldwide. It can manifest in a variety of ways, from chronic worry and restlessness to panic attacks and avoidance behaviors. Left unchecked, anxiety can significantly impact a woman's quality of life, relationships, and overall well-being.

The good news is that Cognitive Behavior Therapy (CBT) offers a range of effective strategies for managing anxiety in women. By identifying anxiety triggers, challenging anxious thoughts, and developing coping skills, women can learn to reduce the frequency and intensity of their anxiety symptoms and live more fulfilling lives.

Before we dive into specific CBT techniques, let's take a closer look at some of the common anxiety triggers and symptoms among women.

One major trigger for anxiety in women is stress related to work, family, and relationships. Women often face unique pressures and expectations in these areas, such as the need to balance career and caregiving responsibilities, the pressure to maintain a certain appearance or body type, and the expectation to be emotionally available and nurturing to others. These stressors can lead to chronic anxiety and feelings of overwhelm.

Another common trigger for anxiety in women is trauma or past experiences of abuse or violence. Women who have experienced sexual assault, domestic violence, or childhood abuse may develop post-traumatic stress disorder (PTSD) or other anxiety disorders as a result. These experiences can lead to feelings of vulnerability, fear, and mistrust, which can persist long after the traumatic event has ended.

Hormonal changes and fluctuations can also contribute to anxiety in women. During menstruation, pregnancy, and menopause, women may experience shifts in mood and energy levels that can trigger anxiety symptoms. Additionally, some women may be more sensitive to hormonal changes due to genetic or environmental factors.

Other common triggers for anxiety in women include health concerns, financial stress, social pressure, and major life transitions such as getting married, having a child, or retiring from work.

So what do anxiety symptoms look like in women? Some common physical symptoms include:
- Racing heartbeat or palpitations
- Sweating or trembling
- Shortness of breath or hyperventilation
- Muscle tension or pain
- Digestive issues such as nausea or diarrhea
- Insomnia or other sleep disturbances

Cognitive symptoms of anxiety may include:
- Chronic worry or rumination
- Difficulty concentrating or making decisions
- Racing or intrusive thoughts
- Feelings of impending danger or doom
- Irritability or restlessness

Behavioral symptoms of anxiety may include:
- Avoidance of certain people, places, or situations
- Compulsive behaviors such as checking or cleaning

- Seeking reassurance from others
- Difficulty asserting oneself or setting boundaries
- Procrastination or perfectionism

It's important to note that anxiety symptoms can vary widely from person to person, and may change over time. Some women may experience primarily physical symptoms, while others may struggle more with cognitive or behavioral symptoms.

Additionally, anxiety disorders can co-occur with other mental health conditions such as depression, substance abuse, or eating disorders. Women with multiple mental health challenges may require a more comprehensive treatment approach that addresses each condition simultaneously.

Now that we have a better understanding of the common triggers and symptoms of anxiety in women, let's explore some CBT techniques for managing anxiety.

One foundational CBT technique is cognitive restructuring, which involves identifying and challenging anxious thoughts. Women with anxiety often have distorted or exaggerated beliefs about themselves, others, and the world around them. These beliefs can fuel anxiety and make it difficult to cope with stressful situations.

For example, a woman with social anxiety may have the belief "Everyone is judging me and thinks I'm awkward." This belief may lead her to avoid social situations or experience intense anxiety when interacting with others. Through cognitive restructuring, she can learn to identify this belief as a cognitive distortion and challenge it with evidence.

She might ask herself questions like:

- What evidence do I have that everyone is judging me negatively?
- Are there any alternative explanations for people's behavior or reactions?
- What would I say to a friend who had this same belief about themselves?

By examining the evidence and considering alternative perspectives, the woman can start to develop a more balanced and realistic view of social situations. She might replace the anxious belief with a more neutral or positive one, such as "Some people may judge me, but most people are probably focused on their own thoughts and experiences."

Cognitive restructuring takes practice and persistence, but over time it can help women develop a more flexible and resilient mindset in the face of anxiety-provoking situations.

Another CBT technique for managing anxiety is relaxation training. When we experience anxiety, our bodies often enter a state of heightened arousal, with increased heart rate, muscle tension, and rapid breathing. Relaxation techniques can help counteract these physical symptoms and promote a sense of calm and well-being.

One common relaxation technique is deep breathing. By taking slow, deep breaths from the diaphragm, women can activate the body's natural relaxation response and reduce feelings of tension and anxiety. To practice deep breathing, women can try the following steps:

1 Find a quiet, comfortable place to sit or lie down.

2 Place one hand on the chest and the other on the belly.

3 Breathe in slowly and deeply through the nose, allowing the belly to expand.

4 Hold the breath for a few seconds, then exhale slowly through the mouth, allowing the belly to fall.

5 Repeat this process for several minutes, focusing on the sensations of the breath entering and leaving the body.

Another relaxation technique is progressive muscle relaxation (PMR). This involves systematically tensing and relaxing different muscle groups in the body to promote overall relaxation and reduce muscle tension. To practice PMR, women can try the following steps:

1 Find a quiet, comfortable place to sit or lie down.

2 Take a few deep breaths and focus on the present moment.

3 Starting with the feet, tense the muscles as tightly as possible for 5-10 seconds.

4 Relax the feet muscles completely and notice the sensation of tension releasing.

5 Move up to the next muscle group (calves, thighs, hips, etc.) and repeat the process of tensing and relaxing.

6 Continue this process until all major muscle groups have been tensed and relaxed.

Relaxation techniques like deep breathing and PMR can be practiced regularly as part of a self-care routine, or used in the moment to cope with acute anxiety symptoms.

A third CBT technique for managing anxiety is exposure therapy. This involves gradually and systematically exposing oneself to feared or avoided situations in order to build tolerance and reduce anxiety over time. Exposure therapy is based on the idea that avoidance of anxiety-provoking situations can actually maintain and worsen anxiety in the long run.

For example, a woman with a phobia of dogs may avoid going to parks or walking in her neighborhood for fear of encountering a dog. Through exposure therapy, she can work with a therapist to develop a hierarchy of increasingly challenging exposures, such as:

1 Looking at pictures of dogs

2 Watching videos of dogs

3 Viewing a dog from a distance in a park

4 Walking past a dog on a leash

5 Petting a friendly dog with the owner's permission

By gradually facing her fear in a controlled and supportive environment, the woman can learn that her anxious predictions (e.g. "the dog will bite me") are unlikely to come true, and that she can cope with the anxiety and discomfort that arise during the exposure.

Exposure therapy can be challenging and may require the guidance of a trained therapist, but it is one of the most effective treatments for anxiety disorders, particularly phobias and social anxiety.

In addition to these specific CBT techniques, there are several general coping strategies that women can use to manage anxiety in their daily lives.

One important strategy is self-care. Women with anxiety often neglect their own needs and well-being in the face of stress and responsibilities. By prioritizing self-care activities such as exercise, healthy eating, sufficient sleep, and enjoyable hobbies, women can build resilience and reduce vulnerability to anxiety.

Another coping strategy is social support. Connecting with friends, family members, or a support group can provide a sense of belonging and validation, and can help women feel less alone in their struggles with anxiety. It's important for women to choose supportive and understanding social connections, and to set boundaries around relationships that may be toxic or draining.

Mindfulness and present-moment awareness can also be helpful for managing anxiety. By focusing on the present moment and accepting one's thoughts and feelings without judgment, women can reduce the power of anxious rumination and worry. Mindfulness practices such as meditation, yoga, or deep breathing can be incorporated into daily life to promote a sense of calm and centeredness.

Finally, it's important for women to challenge perfectionistic or self-critical tendencies that can fuel anxiety. Women with anxiety often hold themselves to unrealistic standards and engage in negative self-talk when they fall short of these standards. By practicing self-compassion and reframing mistakes as opportunities for growth and learning, women can develop a more accepting and resilient relationship with themselves.

In conclusion, managing anxiety through CBT is a powerful and effective approach for women. By identifying anxiety triggers, challenging anxious thoughts, and developing coping skills such as relaxation, exposure, self-care, social support, mindfulness, and self-compassion, women can reduce the impact of anxiety on their lives and cultivate greater well-being and resilience.

It's important to remember that managing anxiety is an ongoing process, and that setbacks and challenges are a normal part of the journey. Women may need to try multiple coping strategies and techniques before finding what works best for them, and may benefit from the support of a therapist or counselor along the way.

At the same time, it's crucial to recognize the strength and courage that it takes to confront anxiety and make positive changes in one's life. Every small step towards greater self-awareness, self-acceptance, and self-care is a victory worth celebrating.

To all the women reading this chapter who struggle with anxiety, know that you are not alone, and that there is hope and help available. You have the power within you to face your fears, challenge your anxious thoughts, and create a life of greater peace, purpose, and joy. May you find the resources, support, and inner wisdom you need to navigate this journey with grace and resilience.

OVERCOMING DEPRESSION WITH CBT: A GUIDE FOR WOMEN

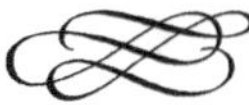

*D*epression is a serious and prevalent mental health challenge that affects millions of women worldwide. It is characterized by persistent feelings of sadness, hopelessness, and a lack of interest or pleasure in daily activities. Depression can have a profound impact on a woman's quality of life, relationships, and overall well-being, making it crucial to recognize the signs and symptoms and seek appropriate treatment.

Women are particularly vulnerable to depression due to a combination of biological, psychological, and social factors. Hormonal changes, such as those experienced during menstrual cycles, pregnancy, and menopause, can contribute to mood fluctuations and increased risk of depression. Additionally, women often face unique stressors and societal pressures, such as juggling multiple roles as caregivers and professionals, experiencing gender-based discrimination or violence, and coping with body image issues and self-esteem challenges.

Recognizing the signs and symptoms of depression is an essential first step in seeking help and support. Some common symptoms of depression in women include:

1 Persistent feelings of sadness, emptiness, or hopelessness

2 Loss of interest or pleasure in activities once enjoyed

3 Significant changes in appetite or weight (either increased or decreased)

4 Sleep disturbances (insomnia or sleeping too much)

5 Fatigue or decreased energy levels

6 Difficulty concentrating, remembering, or making decisions

7 Feelings of worthlessness, guilt, or self-blame

8 Restlessness, irritability, or agitation

9 Physical symptoms such as headaches, digestive issues, or chronic pain

10 Thoughts of death, self-harm, or suicide

It's important to note that not every woman experiences all of these symptoms, and the severity and duration of symptoms can vary from person to person. Some women may experience primarily physical symptoms, while others may struggle more with emotional or cognitive symptoms.

If you or someone you know is experiencing several of these symptoms for more than two weeks, it's crucial to reach out for professional help. Depression is a treatable condition, and early intervention can significantly improve outcomes and prevent the worsening of symptoms.

Cognitive Behavioral Therapy (CBT) is a highly effective treatment approach for managing depression in women. CBT is based on the idea that our thoughts, feelings, and behaviors are interconnected, and that by identifying and changing negative or distorted thought patterns, we can improve our emotional well-being and overall functioning.

One key CBT strategy for managing depression is cognitive restructuring, which involves identifying and challenging negative thoughts and beliefs. Women with depression often have distorted or overly negative views of themselves, their experiences, and their future. These negative thoughts can fuel feelings of hopelessness, worthlessness, and despair, and can make it difficult to engage in positive behaviors or seek support.

For example, a woman with depression might have the thought, "I'm a failure and nothing I do matters." This thought can lead to feelings of sadness and apathy, and may cause her to avoid taking on new challenges or engaging in activities that could improve her mood and self-esteem.

Through cognitive restructuring, the woman can learn to identify this negative thought as a cognitive distortion and challenge it with evidence. She might ask herself questions like:

• What evidence do I have that I'm a complete failure?

• Are there any areas of my life where I have had success or made progress?

• What would I say to a friend who expressed this same thought about themselves?

By examining the evidence and considering alternative perspectives, the woman can start to develop a more balanced and realistic view of herself and her experiences. She might replace the negative thought with a more neutral or compassionate one, such as "I have had both successes and failures in my life, and my worth is not determined by my achievements alone."

Cognitive restructuring takes practice and persistence, but over time it can help women with depression develop a more resilient and adaptive mindset in the face of challenges and setbacks.

Another CBT strategy for managing depression is behavioral activation. When we are depressed, we often lose motivation and interest in activities that once brought us joy and fulfillment. We may withdraw from social connections, neglect self-care, and engage in passive or avoidant behaviors that can worsen our mood and perpetuate the cycle of depression.

Behavioral activation involves deliberately scheduling and engaging in activities that promote a sense of pleasure, mastery, or social connection, even when we don't feel like it. By taking action and challenging our avoidant tendencies, we can gradually improve our mood and build momentum towards recovery.

For example, a woman with depression who has been isolating herself at home might start by setting a small goal of taking a 10-

minute walk outside each day. Even though she may not feel like it, by pushing herself to engage in this simple activity, she can start to experience small moments of pleasure or accomplishment that can boost her mood and motivation.

As she continues to engage in behavioral activation, she can gradually add more challenging or rewarding activities to her schedule, such as:

- Calling a friend or family member for a chat
- Trying a new hobby or creative project
- Volunteering for a cause she cares about
- Attending a support group or social event
- Practicing self-care activities like taking a bath or reading a book

The key is to start small and build up gradually, setting realistic goals and celebrating each step along the way. It's also important to be flexible and adjust the plan as needed based on energy levels, preferences, and life circumstances.

Problem-solving is another valuable CBT strategy for managing depression in women. When we are depressed, we may feel overwhelmed by life's challenges and struggle to find solutions or take action. We may engage in rumination, dwelling on problems without taking steps to address them, which can worsen feelings of hopelessness and despair.

Problem-solving involves breaking down a challenge into smaller, more manageable steps and developing a plan of action. By focusing on what we can control and taking proactive steps towards change, we can build a sense of agency and empowerment, even in the face of difficult circumstances.

For example, a woman with depression who is struggling with financial stress might feel overwhelmed and hopeless about her situation. Through problem-solving, she can break down the challenge into specific, actionable steps, such as:

1 Creating a budget to track income and expenses

2 Identifying areas where she can cut back on spending

3 Exploring options for increasing income, such as taking on a part-time job or freelance work

4 Reaching out to a financial counselor or support service for guidance and resources

5 Communicating with creditors or bill collectors to discuss payment plans or assistance programs

By focusing on these concrete steps, the woman can start to feel a sense of control and progress, even if the overall financial situation remains challenging. Problem-solving can be applied to a wide range of issues, from relationship conflicts to health concerns to career transitions.

In addition to these specific CBT strategies, there are several general coping skills and lifestyle factors that can support women in managing depression.

One important factor is self-care. When we are depressed, we often neglect our physical, emotional, and spiritual needs, which can worsen symptoms and make it harder to recover. By prioritizing self-care activities such as regular exercise, healthy eating, sufficient sleep, and stress management techniques like meditation or deep breathing, we can support our overall well-being and resilience.

It's also crucial for women with depression to cultivate a strong support system. Connecting with trusted friends, family members, or a therapist can provide a sense of validation, belonging, and encouragement. It's important to choose supportive and understanding people who can offer practical and emotional assistance, and to set boundaries around relationships that may be toxic or draining.

Mindfulness and present-moment awareness can also be valuable tools for managing depression. When we are depressed, we often get caught up in negative thoughts about the past or worries about the future, which can fuel feelings of hopelessness and despair. By practicing mindfulness techniques such as meditation, deep breathing, or sensory grounding exercises, we can learn to anchor ourselves in the present moment and observe our thoughts and feelings with greater clarity and objectivity.

Another important factor is finding meaning and purpose in life. When we are depressed, we may struggle to see the value or significance of our experiences and relationships. By reflecting on our values, passions, and goals, and taking steps to align our actions with these priorities, we can cultivate a deeper sense of meaning and direction. This might involve pursuing a meaningful career or volunteer work, nurturing important relationships, or engaging in creative or spiritual practices that bring a sense of fulfillment and joy.

It's also important for women with depression to challenge perfectionistic or self-critical tendencies that can fuel negative self-talk and feelings of inadequacy. Women are often socialized to hold themselves to unrealistic standards of beauty, achievement, and caregiving, and may struggle with feelings of guilt or failure when they fall short of these expectations. By practicing self-compassion and reframing setbacks as opportunities for growth and learning, women can develop a more accepting and resilient relationship with themselves.

Finally, it's crucial for women with depression to be patient and persistent in their recovery journey. Overcoming depression is a gradual process that often involves setbacks and challenges along the way. It's important to celebrate small victories and progress, and to seek additional support or resources when needed.

In some cases, women with depression may benefit from a combination of CBT and medication, such as antidepressants. It's important to work closely with a qualified healthcare provider to determine the best treatment approach based on individual needs and preferences.

In conclusion, overcoming depression through CBT is a powerful and empowering journey for women. By recognizing the signs and symptoms of depression, challenging negative thoughts and beliefs, engaging in behavioral activation and problem-solving, and cultivating self-care, social support, mindfulness, and meaning in life, women can reclaim their sense of agency, resilience, and well-being.

It's important to remember that recovery is possible, and that every woman's journey is unique and valuable. By seeking help and support, practicing self-compassion and persistence, and holding onto hope and purpose, women can emerge from the darkness of depression and build a life of greater joy, connection, and fulfillment.

To all the women reading this chapter who are struggling with depression, know that you are not alone, and that there is hope and help available. You have the strength and courage within you to face this challenge and create a brighter future for yourself and those you love. May you find the resources, support, and inner wisdom you need to navigate this journey with grace and resilience, one day at a time.

ASSERTIVENESS TRAINING AND BOUNDARY SETTING: EMPOWERING WOMEN THROUGH CBT

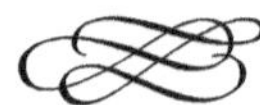

Assertiveness and healthy boundary setting are crucial skills for women's mental health and overall well-being. However, many women struggle with expressing their needs, wants, and limits effectively. This can lead to stress, resentment, burnout, and even more serious mental health issues like depression and anxiety.

In this chapter, we'll explore why assertiveness and boundary setting are so important for women's mental health. We'll also dive into specific Cognitive Behavioral Therapy (CBT) techniques that can help women develop these essential skills and empower themselves in their relationships and daily lives.

Why Assertiveness and Boundary Setting Matter for Women

Assertiveness is the ability to express one's feelings, needs, and beliefs in a clear, direct, and respectful manner. It involves standing up for oneself while also considering the rights and needs of others. Boundary setting, on the other hand, is about defining and communicating the limits of what is acceptable and unacceptable in our relationships and interactions.

For women, assertiveness and boundary setting are particularly important for several reasons:

1 Societal conditioning: From a young age, many girls are taught

to prioritize the needs of others over their own. They may receive messages that it's not feminine or polite to speak up, say no, or assert themselves. This conditioning can lead women to feel guilty, selfish, or uncomfortable when it comes to expressing their own needs and limits.

2 Gender roles and expectations: Women often face pressure to take on nurturing, caregiving roles in their families and communities. They may be expected to be emotionally available, put others' needs first, and maintain harmony in relationships. These expectations can make it difficult for women to set boundaries and prioritize their own self-care and well-being.

3 Power imbalances: In many areas of life, from the workplace to intimate relationships, women may face power imbalances that make assertiveness and boundary setting challenging. They may fear negative consequences like rejection, conflict, or even violence if they speak up or say no.

4 Mental health impact: When women don't feel able to assert their needs and boundaries, it can take a toll on their mental health. They may experience chronic stress, resentment, and burnout from overextending themselves. They may also be more vulnerable to depression, anxiety, and low self-esteem if they feel powerless or unheard in their relationships.

Given these challenges, it's clear that assertiveness and boundary setting are key skills for women to cultivate. But how can women who struggle in these areas build their assertiveness muscles and start setting healthier boundaries? That's where CBT comes in.

CBT Techniques for Developing Assertiveness and Setting Boundaries

Cognitive Behavioral Therapy is a practical, evidence-based approach that helps individuals identify and change unhelpful thought patterns and behaviors. When it comes to assertiveness and boundary setting, CBT offers several powerful techniques:

1 Identifying and challenging unhelpful beliefs: Many women hold beliefs that make assertiveness and boundary setting difficult, such as "I don't have the right to say no," "I'm responsible for everyone else's

feelings," or "Setting boundaries will make people reject me." CBT helps women recognize these beliefs and examine the evidence for and against them. By challenging unhelpful beliefs, women can start to build a more balanced and empowering mindset.

For example, a woman who believes "I don't have the right to say no" might challenge this belief by asking herself:

• Where did I learn this belief? Is it based on facts or societal messages?

• What are the costs of never saying no, to my well-being, relationships, and goals?

• What would I say to a friend who believed she didn't have the right to say no?

Through this process of questioning and reframing, the woman might develop a new belief, such as "I have the right to say no when something doesn't work for me. Saying no allows me to prioritize my well-being and show up more fully in my life."

2 Assertiveness scripts and role-playing: CBT also offers practical tools for building assertiveness skills, such as assertiveness scripts and role-playing exercises. Assertiveness scripts are simple, formula statements that women can use to express their needs, feelings, and boundaries clearly and respectfully.

One common assertiveness script is the "I feel... when... because... I need..." statement. For example:

• "I feel overwhelmed when you ask me to take on extra projects at the last minute, because I already have a full workload. I need at least a week's notice for any additional tasks."

• "I feel hurt when you make jokes about my appearance, because it feels disrespectful. I need you to stop making those kinds of comments."

By practicing assertiveness scripts, women can get more comfortable expressing themselves directly and respectfully. Role-playing exercises, where women practice assertiveness in simulated conversations with a therapist or peer, can also help build confidence and refine communication skills.

3 Boundary setting strategies: CBT also teaches concrete strategies

for setting and maintaining healthy boundaries. One key strategy is learning to say no clearly and firmly, without over-explaining or apologizing. This might sound like:

• "No, I can't take on that extra project this week. Thanks for understanding."

• "No, I'm not comfortable with that level of physical touch. Please respect my boundaries."

Another strategy is learning to communicate boundaries proactively, rather than waiting until they've been crossed. This might involve statements like:

• "Before we dive into this conversation, I want to let you know that I only have 30 minutes to talk today."

• "I'm happy to help out with the kids this weekend, but I'll need some time to myself in the evenings to recharge."

Women can also practice boundary setting in a gradual, step-by-step way, starting with smaller, lower-stakes boundaries and building up to more challenging ones over time. Celebrating successes and learning from setbacks is also key to building boundary-setting confidence.

4 Self-care and emotion regulation: Assertiveness and boundary setting can be emotionally challenging, especially for women who are used to prioritizing others' needs and feelings. That's why CBT also emphasizes the importance of self-care and emotion regulation skills.

Self-care involves intentionally nurturing one's physical, emotional, and mental well-being. This might include activities like regular exercise, getting enough sleep, spending time in nature, engaging in hobbies or creative pursuits, or practicing relaxation techniques like deep breathing or meditation.

Emotion regulation skills help women manage the difficult feelings that can arise when asserting themselves or setting boundaries, such as anxiety, guilt, or self-doubt. These skills might include:

• Naming and validating one's emotions, rather than judging or suppressing them

• Practicing self-compassion and reframing negative self-talk

• Using grounding techniques to stay present and calm in challenging conversations

• Seeking support from trusted friends, family members, or a therapist

By prioritizing self-care and emotion regulation, women can build the resilience and inner resources needed to assert themselves and set boundaries more confidently and consistently.

Putting Assertiveness and Boundary Setting into Practice

While CBT techniques can be powerful tools for building assertiveness and boundary-setting skills, it's important to remember that change takes time and practice. Women may face setbacks, resistance from others, or internal barriers as they start to assert themselves more and set clearer boundaries.

Here are some tips for putting assertiveness and boundary setting into practice in daily life:

1 Start small: Begin practicing assertiveness and boundary setting in low-stakes situations, such as saying no to a salesperson or setting a boundary with a casual acquaintance. Build up gradually to more challenging conversations and relationships.

2 Pick your battles: Assertiveness and boundary setting are important, but it's also okay to choose your battles. Not every minor irritation or request needs to be addressed. Focus on the boundaries and needs that matter most to your well-being and values.

3 Prepare and practice: Before a challenging conversation or boundary-setting moment, take time to prepare. Write down your key points, practice your assertiveness script, and visualize yourself communicating calmly and confidently.

4 Use "I" statements: When expressing your needs and boundaries, focus on your own feelings and experiences, rather than blaming or criticizing others. "I" statements, like "I feel..." or "I need...," can help keep the conversation focused on your perspective.

5 Be willing to compromise: Assertiveness and boundary setting don't mean always getting your way. Be open to finding mutually beneficial solutions and compromises, while still honoring your core needs and limits.

6 Seek support: Surround yourself with supportive people who respect your boundaries and encourage your assertiveness. Consider seeking guidance from a CBT therapist or joining an assertiveness training group for additional support and accountability.

7 Celebrate your successes: Assertiveness and boundary setting are challenging skills to develop, so it's important to celebrate your progress along the way. Acknowledge and appreciate yourself for each step you take towards speaking up for yourself and setting healthier limits.

Real-Life Examples and Stories

To illustrate the power of assertiveness and boundary setting in women's lives, let's explore a few real-life examples and stories.

Example 1: Sarah's work boundaries

Sarah is a 35-year-old graphic designer who often struggles to set boundaries at work. She frequently takes on extra projects and works late into the night, even when it means sacrificing her personal life and well-being. She feels guilty saying no to her boss and colleagues, and worries that setting limits will make her seem uncooperative or underperforming.

Through CBT, Sarah identifies some of the beliefs and patterns that make boundary setting difficult for her, such as:

• "I have to say yes to every request, or I'll be seen as a bad employee."

• "I'm responsible for making sure every project is perfect, even if it means working myself to exhaustion."

• "My own needs and well-being are less important than meeting others' expectations."

Sarah's therapist helps her challenge these beliefs and develop a more balanced perspective. She practices assertiveness scripts like:

• "I appreciate you thinking of me for this project, but my workload is full right now. Can we discuss priorities and timelines to ensure I'm not overextending myself?"

• "I'm happy to help out with that task, but I'll need to leave the office by 6 pm tonight to maintain my work-life balance."

Sarah also starts to prioritize self-care, setting aside time for exercise, hobbies, and relaxation. She communicates her boundaries proactively, such as letting her boss know that she'll be unavailable on weekends and evenings except for true emergencies.

At first, Sarah feels anxious and guilty setting these boundaries. But over time, she notices that her colleagues and boss respect her limits and appreciate her clear communication. She feels more energized, focused, and productive at work, and has more time and energy for her personal life and relationships.

Example 2: Maria's relationship boundaries

Maria is a 28-year-old nurse who has always struggled to assert herself in romantic relationships. She tends to attract partners who are controlling or emotionally unavailable, and finds herself suppressing her own needs and feelings to avoid conflict or rejection.

In her current relationship, Maria's boyfriend often criticizes her appearance, makes plans without consulting her, and dismisses her opinions and concerns. Maria feels increasingly anxious, resentful, and disconnected from herself.

Through CBT, Maria realizes that her difficulty with assertiveness and boundary setting stems from a deep-seated belief that she is unworthy of love and respect. She fears that standing up for herself will lead to abandonment or retaliation.

With her therapist's guidance, Maria begins to challenge this belief and develop a more self-compassionate mindset. She practices assertiveness scripts like:

• "I feel disrespected when you criticize my appearance. I need you to focus on my inner qualities and treat me with kindness."

• "I feel left out when you make plans without asking me. I need to be included in decisions that affect both of us."

Maria also starts to set clearer boundaries around her time, space, and emotional energy. She communicates her needs proactively, such as:

• "I need some alone time this weekend to recharge. Let's plan to spend Saturday together and do our own things on Sunday."

• "I appreciate your advice, but I need to make my own decisions about my career. Please respect my choices."

At first, Maria's boyfriend resists her new assertiveness and boundary setting. But as Maria remains firm and consistent, he begins to adjust his behavior and show more respect for her needs. Maria feels more confident, authentic, and peaceful in the relationship, and is better able to discern whether it aligns with her values and goals.

Example 3: Amy's family boundaries

Amy is a 45-year-old mother of three who has always been the "rock" of her family. She is the one everyone turns to for emotional support, financial help, and caregiving. While Amy loves her family deeply, she often feels overwhelmed, depleted, and resentful.

Amy's adult children frequently drop by unannounced and expect her to babysit at a moment's notice. Her aging parents rely on her for daily check-ins and errands, even though they are still relatively independent. Amy's husband often leaves household tasks and parenting responsibilities to her, assuming she'll handle everything.

Through CBT, Amy realizes that her difficulty with boundary setting stems from a belief that her worth is tied to her ability to care for others. She fears that setting limits will make her a bad mother, daughter, and wife.

Amy's therapist helps her reframe this belief and develop a more balanced perspective. She practices assertiveness scripts like:

• "I love spending time with the grandkids, but I need you to ask me in advance before dropping them off. I have my own commitments and self-care needs."

• "I'm happy to help out with errands, but I can only do so once a week. Let's work together to find other solutions and supports."

Amy also starts to communicate her boundaries and needs more clearly with her husband and children, such as:

• "I need us to share household tasks and parenting responsibilities more evenly. Let's make a plan together."

• "I'm taking a weekend away with friends next month. I trust that you'll be able to handle things here while I'm gone."

At first, Amy's family members are surprised and resistant to her boundary setting. But as Amy remains loving but firm, they start to adjust and respect her limits. Amy's children and parents find more independence and resilience, and her husband steps up to share the load at home.

Amy begins to feel more balanced, fulfilled, and appreciated in her family roles. She has more energy and joy for the caregiving she chooses to do, and more time for her own self-care and interests. Her relationships with her family members become more mutual and sustainable.

From these examples, we can see how assertiveness and boundary setting can transform women's lives and relationships. By challenging limiting beliefs, practicing clear communication, and prioritizing self-care, women can empower themselves to create more balanced, fulfilling, and authentic lives.

Conclusion

In conclusion, assertiveness and boundary setting are essential skills for women's mental health and well-being. By learning to express their needs, wants, and limits clearly and confidently, women can reduce stress, build healthier relationships, and cultivate a stronger sense of self.

Cognitive Behavioral Therapy offers a range of powerful tools and techniques for developing assertiveness and boundary-setting skills, including:

1 Identifying and challenging unhelpful beliefs

2 Practicing assertiveness scripts and role-playing

3 Implementing specific boundary-setting strategies

4 Prioritizing self-care and emotion regulation

While developing assertiveness and boundary-setting skills takes time, practice, and patience, the benefits are well worth the effort. As women become more empowered to speak up for themselves and set healthy limits, they can experience greater peace, joy, and fulfillment in all areas of their lives.

If you're a woman struggling with assertiveness and boundary setting, know that you're not alone. Seeking support from a CBT therapist, assertiveness training group, or supportive friends and family can make a world of difference. With practice, self-compassion, and a commitment to your own well-being, you can develop the skills and confidence to create the life and relationships you truly desire.

Remember, assertiveness and boundary setting are not about being selfish or uncaring. They are about honoring your own needs and limits so that you can show up more fully and authentically in your life and relationships. By empowering yourself to speak your truth and set healthy boundaries, you inspire others to do the same. You create a ripple effect of positive change that benefits everyone around you.

So take a deep breath, trust in your own strength and wisdom, and start taking small, consistent steps towards assertiveness and boundary setting today. Your mental health, relationships, and overall well-being will thank you.

NAVIGATING RELATIONSHIPS WITH CBT: STRATEGIES FOR WOMEN

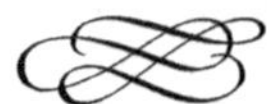

*R*elationships are a central part of most women's lives, providing connection, support, and meaning. However, relationships can also be a source of stress, conflict, and emotional pain, particularly when negative thought patterns and low self-esteem are at play.

In this chapter, we'll explore how Cognitive Behavioral Therapy (CBT) can help women navigate the complexities of relationships, from friendships and family dynamics to romantic partnerships and professional connections. We'll look at how negative thought patterns and low self-esteem can impact relationships, and provide specific CBT techniques for improving communication, resolving conflicts, and building healthier, more fulfilling relationships.

The Impact of Negative Thought Patterns on Relationships

Negative thought patterns, also known as cognitive distortions, are habitual ways of thinking that are often exaggerated, irrational, or inaccurate. These thought patterns can have a profound impact on how we perceive and interact with others, leading to misunderstandings, conflicts, and relational dissatisfaction.

Some common negative thought patterns that can affect relationships include:

1 Mind reading: This involves assuming we know what others are thinking or feeling, without checking for accuracy. For example, a woman might assume her partner is annoyed with her because he's been quiet all evening, when in reality he's just tired from a long day at work.

2 Fortune telling: This involves predicting negative outcomes in relationships, often without evidence. For example, a woman might believe that every romantic relationship she enters is doomed to fail, based on past experiences of heartbreak.

3 All-or-nothing thinking: This involves seeing situations in black-and-white terms, without acknowledging nuance or complexity. For example, a woman might believe that if her friend cancels plans with her once, it means the friend doesn't care about her at all.

4 Overgeneralization: This involves drawing broad conclusions based on a single incident or piece of evidence. For example, a woman might have one negative interaction with a colleague and conclude that the entire workplace is hostile and unfriendly.

5 Personalization: This involves taking things personally and assuming blame for events that are outside of one's control. For example, a woman might believe that her child's misbehavior is a direct reflection of her parenting skills, even when other factors are at play.

When these negative thought patterns are left unchecked, they can lead to a range of relational problems. Women may feel anxious, insecure, or resentful in their connections with others. They may avoid intimacy or vulnerability for fear of rejection or betrayal. They may engage in self-sabotaging behaviors, such as picking fights or pushing others away.

The Impact of Low Self-Esteem on Relationships

Low self-esteem, or a negative overall view of oneself, can also have a significant impact on women's relationships. When women don't feel worthy of love, respect, and care, they may settle for less than they deserve in their connections with others.

Some ways that low self-esteem can manifest in relationships include:

1 People-pleasing: Women with low self-esteem may go out of their way to please others and avoid conflict, even when it means sacrificing their own needs and boundaries. They may say yes to requests they don't want to fulfill, or apologize excessively for minor mistakes.

2 Difficulty with assertiveness: Women with low self-esteem may struggle to express their thoughts, feelings, and needs directly and respectfully. They may use passive or aggressive communication styles, or avoid speaking up altogether.

3 Tolerance of mistreatment: Women with low self-esteem may tolerate disrespect, neglect, or even abuse in their relationships, believing they don't deserve better treatment. They may make excuses for their partner's behavior or blame themselves for relational problems.

4 Excessive jealousy or possessiveness: Women with low self-esteem may feel threatened by their partner's independence or outside relationships, fearing abandonment or betrayal. They may engage in controlling or possessive behaviors in an attempt to keep their partner close.

5 Negative self-talk: Women with low self-esteem may engage in harsh, critical self-talk that undermines their confidence and worth in relationships. They may compare themselves unfavorably to others or dismiss their own strengths and accomplishments.

When low self-esteem and negative thought patterns combine, they can create a perfect storm of relational challenges. Women may feel trapped in unfulfilling or even toxic relationships, believing they have no other options or deserve nothing better.

The good news is that CBT offers a range of strategies and techniques for overcoming negative thought patterns, building self-esteem, and improving relational dynamics. By learning to identify and challenge cognitive distortions, communicate effectively, and set healthy boundaries, women can cultivate more loving, respectful, and satisfying relationships with others and with themselves.

CBT Techniques for Improving Communication

Effective communication is the foundation of any healthy relationship, whether with a romantic partner, family member, friend, or colleague. However, many women struggle with communication skills, particularly when negative thought patterns or low self-esteem are at play.

CBT offers several techniques for improving communication and building stronger, more authentic connections:

1 Active listening: This involves giving your full attention to the other person, without interrupting, judging, or planning your response. Active listening requires putting aside your own agenda temporarily and focusing on understanding the other person's perspective.

Some tips for active listening include:

• Make eye contact and use open, receptive body language

• Paraphrase or summarize what the other person has said to ensure understanding

• Ask clarifying questions to gather more information

• Validate the other person's feelings, even if you disagree with their perspective

Active listening helps build trust, empathy, and connection in relationships. When women feel truly heard and understood by others, they are more likely to open up and share their own thoughts and feelings.

2 "I" statements: This technique involves expressing your own thoughts, feelings, and needs directly and respectfully, without blaming or attacking the other person. "I" statements typically follow the formula: "I feel [emotion] when [situation], because [reason]. I would like [request]."

For example:

• "I feel frustrated when you leave dishes in the sink, because I end up having to clean them myself. I would like us to come up with a system for sharing household chores more evenly."

• "I feel hurt when you cancel our plans at the last minute, because it makes me feel unimportant. I would like us to communicate more clearly about our availability and commitments."

Using "I" statements helps reduce defensiveness and promote

open, honest dialogue. It allows women to take ownership of their own experiences and express their needs assertively, without resorting to criticism or demands.

3 Nonviolent communication: This approach, developed by psychologist Marshall Rosenberg, emphasizes the importance of expressing oneself honestly and receiving others' messages with empathy. Nonviolent communication involves four key steps: a. Observation: Describing what you observe without judgment or evaluation. b. Feeling: Expressing your emotions clearly and directly. c. Need: Identifying the underlying need or value that is driving your feelings. d. Request: Making a specific, actionable request of the other person.

For example:

• "When I see clothes on the floor (observation), I feel frustrated (feeling) because I have a need for order and cleanliness (need). Would you be willing to put your clothes in the hamper when you take them off (request)?"

Nonviolent communication helps create a safe, respectful space for both parties to express themselves and work towards mutually satisfying solutions. It encourages women to take responsibility for their own experiences and needs, while also acknowledging the humanity and needs of others.

4 Assertiveness training: As we explored in the previous chapter, assertiveness is the ability to express one's thoughts, feelings, and needs directly and respectfully, without aggression or passivity. Assertiveness training can help women communicate more effectively in their relationships, particularly when setting boundaries or navigating conflicts.

Some key assertiveness skills include:

• Using clear, concise language

• Maintaining open, confident body language and tone of voice

• Practicing "broken record" technique, calmly repeating your message until heard

• Disengaging from unproductive arguments or attacks

• Reinforcing your message with action, such as leaving a conversation or setting a consequence

Assertiveness allows women to advocate for themselves and their relationships in a healthy, proactive way. It helps them feel more in control of their own experiences and less at the mercy of others' actions or opinions.

By practicing active listening, "I" statements, nonviolent communication, and assertiveness skills, women can improve the quality and depth of their relationships. They can foster greater understanding, respect, and collaboration with others, leading to more fulfilling connections and a stronger sense of self.

CBT Techniques for Resolving Conflicts

Conflicts are a normal and inevitable part of any relationship. However, when conflicts are handled poorly, they can lead to resentment, disconnection, and even the dissolution of relationships.

CBT offers several techniques for resolving conflicts constructively and compassionately:

1 Identifying cognitive distortions: As we explored earlier, negative thought patterns can fuel relational conflicts by leading to misinterpretations, assumptions, and reactive behaviors. By learning to identify and challenge these cognitive distortions, women can approach conflicts with greater clarity and objectivity.

For example, a woman who tends to personalize her partner's behavior might have the following internal dialogue during a conflict:

• Automatic thought: "He's being cold and distant because he doesn't love me anymore."

• Challenging questions: "Is there any evidence that his behavior is about me personally? Could there be other factors, like stress at work, contributing to his mood? How would I respond to a friend in this situation?"

• Alternative thought: "His distance may feel hurtful, but it's likely not a reflection of his feelings for me. I can express my own feelings and needs without making assumptions about his intentions."

By challenging cognitive distortions, women can reduce the intensity of conflicts and approach problem-solving with a more balanced, rational mindset.

2 Collaborative problem-solving: This technique involves working with the other person to find mutually satisfying solutions to conflicts. Collaborative problem-solving requires setting aside blame and defensiveness and focusing on the underlying needs and goals of both parties.

The steps of collaborative problem-solving include: a. Defining the problem clearly and objectively b. Brainstorming potential solutions without judgment c. Evaluating the pros and cons of each solution d. Choosing a solution that meets both parties' needs e. Implementing the solution and assessing its effectiveness

For example, a couple struggling with different sleep schedules might engage in the following problem-solving dialogue:

• Problem: "We have different sleep needs that are causing friction in our relationship."

• Brainstorming: "We could go to bed at the same time, even if one of us isn't tired. We could sleep in separate rooms. We could find a compromise bedtime that works for both of us."

• Evaluating: "Going to bed at the same time every night might lead to resentment and sleep deprivation. Sleeping in separate rooms could feel disconnecting. Finding a compromise bedtime seems like the most viable option."

• Choosing: "Let's try going to bed at 10pm on weeknights and 11pm on weekends. We can reassess in a month and make adjustments as needed."

Collaborative problem-solving helps build trust, respect, and a sense of partnership in relationships. It allows both parties to feel heard and validated, while also working towards practical, mutually beneficial solutions.

3 Time-outs and breaks: When conflicts become heated or unproductive, it can be helpful to take a break and return to the discussion when both parties are calmer and more centered. Time-outs can prevent the escalation of conflicts and allow for reflection and perspective-taking.

Some guidelines for effective time-outs include:

• Agreeing on a time-out signal or phrase beforehand, such as "I need a break"

• Specifying a time to return to the discussion, such as "Let's take 20 minutes and come back to this"

• Using the break to engage in self-care activities, such as deep breathing, meditation, or a walk outside

• Avoiding rumination or rehearsal of arguments during the break

• Returning to the discussion with a solutions-focused mindset

Time-outs can be particularly helpful for women who tend to become emotionally flooded or reactive during conflicts. They provide an opportunity to self-soothe, gather thoughts, and approach the discussion with greater intentionality and care.

4 Repair attempts: Even with the best communication and problem-solving skills, conflicts can sometimes lead to hurt feelings, misunderstandings, or disconnection. Repair attempts are efforts to restore connection and goodwill after a conflict or rupture.

Repair attempts can take many forms, such as:

• Offering a sincere apology

• Expressing empathy or understanding for the other person's perspective

• Making a kind gesture, such as a hug, a thoughtful note, or a favorite meal

• Engaging in a shared activity or inside joke

• Reaffirming your commitment to the relationship and its future

Repair attempts help build resilience and trust in relationships. They communicate that conflicts and mistakes are inevitable, but the relationship is worth working through them. When women can offer and receive repair attempts gracefully, they create a sense of emotional safety and continuity in their connections.

By practicing cognitive restructuring, collaborative problem-solving, time-outs, and repair attempts, women can navigate relational conflicts with greater skill and compassion. They can use conflicts as opportunities for growth, understanding, and intimacy, rather than sources of disconnection or pain.

CBT Techniques for Building Healthier Relationships

Beyond improving communication and resolving conflicts, CBT also offers techniques for building healthier, more fulfilling relationships overall. These techniques focus on developing a strong sense of self, setting appropriate boundaries, and cultivating positive relational habits.

1 Self-validation: This involves learning to affirm and accept one's own thoughts, feelings, and needs, rather than relying on others for validation. Self-validation is particularly important for women who tend to base their self-worth on others' approval or acceptance.

Some techniques for self-validation include:

• Practicing self-compassion and kind self-talk

• Keeping a journal of accomplishments, strengths, and positive qualities

• Developing a robust sense of identity and purpose outside of relationships

• Seeking feedback and support from trusted friends, family, or a therapist

• Celebrating personal milestones and successes

Self-validation helps women feel more secure and self-assured in their relationships. When they can affirm their own worth and value, they are less likely to tolerate mistreatment, settle for less than they deserve, or lose themselves in their connections with others.

2 Boundary-setting: As we explored in the previous chapter, boundaries are essential for healthy relationships. They communicate what is and is not acceptable in terms of treatment, time, energy, and resources.

Some tips for effective boundary-setting include:

• Identifying your own needs, limits, and dealbreakers

• Communicating boundaries clearly, calmly, and consistently

• Following through with consequences when boundaries are violated

• Seeking support from others when enforcing difficult boundaries

• Regularly reassessing and adjusting boundaries as needed

Boundary-setting helps women maintain a sense of autonomy, respect, and control in their relationships. It prevents resentment, burnout, and imbalanced power dynamics, and allows for healthier, more mutual connections.

3 Gratitude and appreciation: Expressing gratitude and appreciation is a powerful way to strengthen and deepen relationships. It involves regularly acknowledging and expressing thanks for the positive qualities, actions, and contributions of others.

Some ways to cultivate gratitude and appreciation in relationships include:

• Keeping a gratitude journal and noting specific things you appreciate about your loved ones

• Expressing appreciation verbally, through words of affirmation or praise

• Showing appreciation through acts of service, thoughtful gestures, or quality time

• Practicing mindfulness and savoring positive relationship moments

• Expressing gratitude for challenges and conflicts as opportunities for growth

Gratitude and appreciation help shift the focus in relationships from negativity and criticism to positivity and connection. They build a culture of mutual respect, admiration, and goodwill, and help buffer against stress and conflict.

4 Shared activities and rituals: Engaging in shared activities and rituals is a powerful way to build connection, intimacy, and a sense of partnership in relationships. These can be as simple as a daily check-in conversation or as elaborate as an annual vacation tradition.

Some ideas for shared activities and rituals include:

• Cooking or trying new restaurants together

• Engaging in a shared hobby or interest, such as hiking, dancing, or reading

• Volunteering or engaging in community service together

• Creating a regular date night or quality time ritual

• Developing a shared vision or goal for the relationship, such as saving for a house or planning a trip

Shared activities and rituals help create a sense of unity, purpose, and enjoyment in relationships. They provide opportunities for bonding, laughter, and the creation of positive memories, and can help reignite connection and intimacy during times of stress or distance.

By practicing self-validation, boundary-setting, gratitude and appreciation, and shared activities and rituals, women can build healthier, more fulfilling relationships with others. These techniques help create a strong foundation of self-worth, mutual respect, and shared meaning, which can weather the inevitable ups and downs of relational life.

Real-Life Examples and Stories

To illustrate the power of CBT techniques for navigating relationships, let's explore a few real-life examples and stories.

Example 1: Sarah and John's communication breakthrough

Sarah and John have been married for ten years and have two young children. They love each other deeply, but often struggle with communication and conflict. Sarah tends to bottle up her feelings and withdraw when upset, while John tends to become defensive and argumentative.

SELF-CARE AND STRESS MANAGEMENT: A CBT APPROACH FOR WOMEN

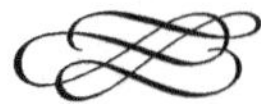

In today's fast-paced, high-pressure world, self-care and stress management are more important than ever for maintaining mental health and well-being. This is especially true for women, who often juggle multiple roles and responsibilities, such as work, family, and caregiving, while also facing unique stressors such as gender discrimination and societal pressures.

However, many women struggle with prioritizing self-care and managing stress effectively. They may view self-care as selfish or indulgent, or feel guilty for taking time away from their many obligations. They may also lack the tools and strategies for coping with stress in healthy and productive ways.

The good news is that Cognitive Behavioral Therapy (CBT) offers a practical, evidence-based approach to self-care and stress management that can help women enhance their mental health, prevent burnout, and improve their overall quality of life. By identifying and challenging unhelpful thoughts and beliefs about self-care, developing personalized self-care plans, and practicing specific stress-reduction techniques, women can cultivate greater resilience, balance, and joy in their lives.

The Importance of Self-Care for Women's Mental Health

Self-care refers to the practices and activities that we engage in to promote our physical, emotional, and mental well-being. It involves taking intentional steps to nurture and support ourselves, so that we can show up more fully and effectively in our lives and relationships.

For women, self-care is particularly important for several reasons:

1 Prevention of burnout: Women are at higher risk for burnout than men, due to the many demands and expectations placed on them both at work and at home. Burnout is a state of physical, emotional, and mental exhaustion caused by chronic stress and overwork. It can lead to a range of negative consequences, such as decreased productivity, increased absenteeism, strained relationships, and even serious health problems like heart disease and depression.

By engaging in regular self-care practices, women can prevent or mitigate the effects of burnout. Self-care helps to reduce stress, replenish energy levels, and promote a sense of balance and well-being, which can buffer against the negative impacts of chronic stress.

2 Enhancement of physical health: Self-care practices such as regular exercise, healthy eating, and sufficient sleep are essential for maintaining physical health and preventing chronic diseases. For women, self-care can be especially important for managing physical health concerns such as menstrual and menopausal symptoms, pregnancy and postpartum recovery, and age-related changes.

By prioritizing self-care, women can improve their physical health outcomes and quality of life. They may experience benefits such as increased energy levels, better sleep, reduced pain and inflammation, and lower risk of chronic diseases such as obesity, diabetes, and heart disease.

3 Promotion of emotional well-being: Self-care practices such as therapy, journaling, and social connection can be powerful tools for promoting emotional well-being and managing mental health concerns such as anxiety, depression, and trauma. For women, who are more likely than men to experience these concerns, self-care can be a vital component of treatment and recovery.

By engaging in self-care practices that promote emotional processing, self-reflection, and healthy coping, women can build greater resilience and self-awareness. They may experience benefits such as improved mood, increased self-esteem, healthier relationships, and greater overall life satisfaction.

4 Role modeling for others: When women prioritize self-care, they not only benefit themselves but also set a positive example for others in their lives, such as children, partners, and colleagues. By demonstrating the value and importance of self-care, women can help to create a culture of well-being and self-compassion that benefits everyone.

This is especially important for mothers, who play a key role in shaping their children's attitudes and behaviors around self-care. When children see their mothers taking care of themselves and managing stress in healthy ways, they are more likely to develop these habits themselves and carry them into adulthood.

Despite the clear benefits of self-care, many women struggle to make it a priority in their lives. They may face barriers such as lack of time, financial resources, or support from others. They may also hold beliefs or attitudes that make self-care challenging, such as:
- "Self-care is selfish or indulgent."
- "I don't deserve to take time for myself."
- "I have to put others' needs before my own."
- "I should be able to handle stress on my own."
- "Self-care is a luxury, not a necessity."

These beliefs can lead women to neglect their own needs and well-being, and to experience the negative consequences of chronic stress and burnout.

The CBT approach to self-care challenges these unhelpful beliefs and provides practical strategies for overcoming barriers to self-care. By developing a personalized self-care plan and practicing specific stress-reduction techniques, women can learn to prioritize their own well-being and experience the many benefits of self-care for mental and physical health.

Developing a Personalized Self-Care Plan

One of the key components of the CBT approach to self-care is developing a personalized self-care plan. This involves identifying specific self-care practices that are enjoyable, feasible, and effective for promoting well-being, and creating a plan for incorporating them into daily life.

Here are some steps for developing a personalized self-care plan:

1 Assess your current self-care practices: Take some time to reflect on your current self-care practices, both positive and negative. Consider questions such as:

- What self-care practices do I currently engage in, if any?
- What practices do I find most enjoyable and effective?
- What practices do I struggle with or avoid?
- What barriers or challenges do I face in practicing self-care?

2 Identify your self-care needs and preferences: Think about what you need to feel your best, both physically and emotionally. Consider factors such as:

- Physical needs: exercise, nutrition, sleep, rest, medical care
- Emotional needs: social connection, creative expression, relaxation, fun
- Spiritual needs: meditation, prayer, time in nature, volunteering
- Intellectual needs: learning, reading, engaging in hobbies or interests

3 Brainstorm self-care ideas: Generate a list of potential self-care practices that align with your needs and preferences. Be creative and think outside the box! Some ideas might include:

- Taking a daily walk or bike ride
- Practicing yoga or meditation
- Cooking healthy meals or trying new recipes
- Engaging in a creative hobby like painting, writing, or music
- Scheduling regular social activities with friends or family
- Taking a relaxing bath or practicing self-massage
- Attending a support group or therapy session
- Taking breaks throughout the workday to stretch or practice deep breathing

4 Create a realistic plan: Once you have a list of potential self-care practices, it's time to create a realistic plan for incorporating them into your daily life. Consider factors such as:

○ Time: How much time can you realistically dedicate to self-care each day or week?

○ Resources: What resources (financial, material, social) do you need to engage in your chosen practices?

○ Barriers: What barriers or challenges might you face in implementing your plan, and how can you address them?

○ Support: Who can you enlist to support you in your self-care efforts, such as a partner, friend, or therapist?

5 Implement and adjust your plan: Once you have created your self-care plan, it's time to put it into action! Start small and build up gradually, rather than trying to overhaul your entire lifestyle overnight. Be patient and compassionate with yourself as you develop new habits and routines.

Regularly assess how your plan is working for you, and make adjustments as needed. You may find that certain practices are more or less effective than you anticipated, or that your needs and preferences change over time. Be flexible and open to experimentation as you fine-tune your self-care plan.

Here's a sample self-care plan to illustrate this process:

• Morning: 10-minute meditation and stretching routine before work

• Midday: 30-minute walk or exercise break, healthy lunch with a colleague or friend

• Evening: 30 minutes of creative hobby or relaxation activity, such as reading or knitting

• Weekly: One social activity with friends or family, one therapy or support group session

• Monthly: One self-care "treat" or indulgence, such as a massage or weekend getaway

Remember, your self-care plan should be personalized to your unique needs, preferences, and circumstances. What works for someone else may not work for you, and that's okay. The key is to find a self-care routine that feels sustainable, enjoyable, and effective for promoting your own well-being.

CBT Techniques for Managing Stress

In addition to developing a personalized self-care plan, CBT also offers specific techniques for managing stress in the moment. These techniques can be particularly helpful for women who face chronic or acute stressors, such as workplace demands, family conflicts, or health concerns.

Here are some CBT techniques for managing stress:

1 Cognitive restructuring: This technique involves identifying and challenging the unhelpful thoughts and beliefs that contribute to stress. When we're stressed, we often engage in negative self-talk or catastrophic thinking, which can exacerbate our distress and make it harder to cope.

Cognitive restructuring helps us to reframe these thoughts in a more balanced and realistic way. For example:

• Stressful thought: "I'll never be able to handle this project on top of everything else I have going on."

• Reframe: "This project is challenging, but I have handled difficult tasks before. I can break it down into smaller steps and ask for support if I need it."

By challenging our negative thoughts and replacing them with more realistic and empowering ones, we can reduce our stress levels and increase our sense of control and efficacy.

2 Relaxation techniques: Relaxation techniques are designed to help us calm our bodies and minds in the face of stress. When we're stressed, our bodies often enter a state of "fight or flight," character-ized by increased heart rate, rapid breathing, and muscle tension. Relaxation techniques help to counteract these physiological responses and promote a sense of calm and well-being.

Some common relaxation techniques include:

• Deep breathing: Taking slow, deep breaths from the diaphragm can help to reduce tension and promote relaxation. Try inhaling for a count of four, holding for a count of four, and exhaling for a count of four.

• Progressive muscle relaxation: This technique involves systemat-ically tensing and releasing different muscle groups in the body, starting with the toes and working up to the head. By consciously releasing tension in the body, we can signal to the mind that it's safe to relax.

• Guided imagery: This technique involves using mental imagery to create a sense of calm and relaxation. You might imagine yourself in a peaceful setting, such as a beach or a forest, and engage all of your senses to fully immerse yourself in the experience.

• Mindfulness meditation: This technique involves focusing your attention on the present moment, without judgment or distraction. By observing your thoughts and sensations with curiosity and acceptance, you can cultivate a sense of inner peace and stability.

3 Time management strategies: Many women experience stress due to feeling overwhelmed by their many responsibilities and obligations. Time management strategies can help to reduce this sense of overwhelm and increase feelings of control and productivity.

Some effective time management strategies include:

• Prioritization: Identify your most important tasks and responsibilities, and focus on these first. Use tools like the Eisenhower Matrix to help you prioritize based on urgency and importance.

• Delegation: Look for tasks or responsibilities that can be delegated to others, such as family members, colleagues, or hired help. Letting go of the need to do everything yourself can be a powerful stress-reliever.

• Scheduling: Use a planner or calendar to schedule your tasks and activities, including self-care practices. Be realistic about how much time each task will take, and build in buffer time for unexpected challenges or interruptions.

• Boundaries: Set clear boundaries around your time and energy, and communicate these to others. Learn to say "no" to requests or invitations that don't align with your priorities or self-care needs.

4 Lifestyle factors: In addition to specific stress-management techniques, CBT also emphasizes the importance of overall lifestyle factors in reducing stress and promoting well-being. These factors include:

○ Exercise: Regular physical activity has been shown to reduce stress, improve mood, and promote overall health and well-being.

Aim for at least 30 minutes of moderate exercise most days of the week, such as brisk walking, cycling, or swimming.

o Nutrition: Eating a balanced, nutrient-rich diet can help to support physical and mental health and reduce the negative impacts of stress. Focus on whole foods like fruits, vegetables, whole grains, and lean proteins, and limit processed and high-sugar foods.

o Sleep: Getting enough quality sleep is essential for managing stress and promoting overall well-being. Aim for 7-9 hours of sleep per night, and practice good sleep hygiene habits like establishing a regular sleep schedule, creating a relaxing bedtime routine, and avoiding screens before bed.

o Social support: Strong social connections and support can buffer against the negative effects of stress and promote resilience. Make time for meaningful connections with friends, family, and community, and don't hesitate to reach out for help when needed.

By incorporating these CBT techniques and lifestyle factors into your self-care plan, you can develop a comprehensive approach to stress management that promotes long-term mental and physical well-being.

Real-Life Examples and Tips

To illustrate how these CBT techniques can be applied in real life, let's look at some examples and tips:

Example 1: Sarah's self-care plan

Sarah is a busy working mother of two who has been feeling overwhelmed and stressed lately. She realizes that she has been neglecting her own self-care needs in favor of taking care of her family and job responsibilities.

Using the CBT approach, Sarah develops the following self-care plan:

• Morning: Wake up 30 minutes earlier for a quick yoga or meditation practice

• Midday: Take a 10-minute walk outside during lunch break, pack a healthy lunch from home

• Evening: Spend 30 minutes on a relaxing activity like reading or knitting, limit screen time before bed

• Weekly: Schedule one social activity with friends, such as a coffee date or yoga class

• Monthly: Take a half-day off work for a self-care activity, such as a massage or nature hike

Sarah also identifies some common cognitive distortions that contribute to her stress, such as "I should be able to handle everything on my own" and "I'm a bad mom if I take time for myself." She practices reframing these thoughts in a more balanced way, such as "It's okay to ask for help and support" and "Taking care of myself makes me a better mom."

By implementing her self-care plan and challenging her negative thoughts, Sarah begins to feel more balanced, energized, and resilient in the face of stress.

Example 2: Maria's stress-management toolbox

Maria is a college student who struggles with anxiety and stress, particularly around exams and deadlines. She often finds herself feeling overwhelmed and paralyzed by her coursework, and has difficulty concentrating and sleeping.

Using CBT techniques, Maria develops the following stress-management toolbox:

• Deep breathing: When she feels her anxiety rising, Maria takes a few minutes to practice deep, diaphragmatic breathing, inhaling for a count of four and exhaling for a count of six.

• Progressive muscle relaxation: Before bed, Maria practices tensing and releasing each muscle group in her body, starting with her toes and working up to her head. This helps her to release physical tension and promote better sleep.

• Time management: Maria uses a planner to break down her assignments into smaller, manageable tasks and schedule them throughout the week. She also sets realistic goals and timelines for each task, and builds in buffer time for unexpected challenges.

• Self-care breaks: Maria schedules regular self-care breaks throughout her day, such as taking a quick walk outside, listening to a favorite song, or calling a friend for support. These breaks help her to recharge and refocus, and prevent burnout.

By using these tools consistently, Maria finds that she is better able to manage her anxiety and stress, and feels more confident and capable in her academic pursuits.

Tips for Success:

1 Start small: When developing a self-care plan or stress-management toolbox, start with small, achievable goals and practices. Don't try to overhaul your entire life overnight, as this can be overwhelming and unsustainable. Instead, focus on making gradual, incremental changes that feel manageable and enjoyable.

2 Be consistent: Consistency is key when it comes to self-care and stress management. Try to incorporate your chosen practices into your daily or weekly routine, and make them a non-negotiable part of your schedule. The more consistently you practice self-care and stress management, the more benefits you will experience over time.

3 Be flexible: While consistency is important, it's also important to be flexible and adaptable. Life is unpredictable, and there will be times when your usual self-care or stress-management practices are not possible or practical. In these moments, be willing to adjust your plans and find alternative ways to care for yourself, such as taking a quick stretch break at your desk or practicing a few minutes of deep breathing.

4 Seek support: Self-care and stress management are not solo endeavors. Seek out support from friends, family, or professionals who can encourage and motivate you in your efforts. Consider joining a support group or working with a therapist who specializes in CBT and stress management.

5 Celebrate your successes: Finally, don't forget to celebrate your successes and progress along the way. Acknowledge and appreciate the small victories, such as taking a daily walk or practicing a relaxation technique before bed. These small steps can add up to big changes over time, and celebrating them can help to reinforce your commitment and motivation.

Conclusion

In conclusion, self-care and stress management are essential components of mental health and well-being for women. By developing a personalized self-care plan, practicing specific stress-reduction techniques, and incorporating healthy lifestyle factors, women can cultivate greater resilience, balance, and joy in their lives.

The CBT approach offers a practical, evidence-based framework for self-care and stress management that can be tailored to each woman's unique needs, preferences, and circumstances. By identifying and challenging unhelpful thoughts and beliefs about self-care, and replacing them with more balanced and empowering ones, women can overcome barriers to self-care and prioritize their own well-being.

Some key takeaways from this chapter include:

1 Self-care is not selfish or indulgent, but rather a necessary component of mental and physical health. By taking care of ourselves, we are better able to show up fully and effectively in our lives and relationships.

2 Developing a personalized self-care plan involves assessing our current practices, identifying our needs and preferences, brainstorming ideas, creating a realistic plan, and implementing and adjusting it over time.

3 CBT techniques for managing stress include cognitive restructuring, relaxation techniques, time management strategies, and lifestyle factors such as exercise, nutrition, sleep, and social support.

4 Consistency, flexibility, support, and celebration are all important factors in successful self-care and stress management.

5 By prioritizing self-care and stress management, women can prevent burnout, enhance physical health, promote emotional well-being, and role model healthy habits for others.

Remember, self-care and stress management are ongoing practices, not one-time events. It's normal to face challenges and setbacks along the way, and to need to adjust and adapt your practices over time. The key is to approach self-care and stress management with compassion, curiosity, and a willingness to experiment and learn.

As women, we often face unique stressors and pressures that can make self-care and stress management feel challenging or even impossible at times. But by making self-care a non-negotiable priority, and using CBT techniques to manage stress and cultivate resilience, we can empower ourselves to thrive in the face of life's challenges and demands.

So start small, be consistent, and don't be afraid to ask for help and support along the way. Your mental and physical health are worth investing in, and the benefits of self-care and stress management will ripple out into all areas of your life.

To all the women reading this chapter, know that you are worthy of self-care and self-compassion, and that prioritizing your own well-being is not only necessary, but transformative. By taking small, consistent steps towards self-care and stress management, you are planting the seeds for a healthier, happier, and more fulfilling life. Keep going, and remember that you are not alone on this journey.

MAINTAINING PROGRESS AND PREVENTING RELAPSE: LONG-TERM CBT STRATEGIES FOR WOMEN

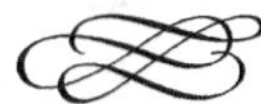

*C*ongratulations on making it to the final chapter of this book! If you've been following along and implementing the strategies and techniques discussed in the previous chapters, you've likely made significant progress in your personal growth and mental well-being. However, it's important to remember that the work doesn't end here. Maintaining the gains you've made through Cognitive Behavioral Therapy (CBT) and preventing relapse is an ongoing process that requires commitment, self-awareness, and a proactive approach.

In this chapter, we'll explore the importance of maintaining progress and preventing relapse, and provide you with practical, long-term CBT strategies to help you continue your personal growth and empowerment journey beyond the initial CBT work. We'll discuss the common challenges and obstacles that women may face in maintaining their progress, and offer tips and techniques for overcoming these hurdles. By the end of this chapter, you'll have a solid understanding of how to integrate CBT principles into your daily life, build resilience, and continue to thrive in the face of life's challenges.

Why Maintaining Progress and Preventing Relapse is Crucial

Picture this: You've been working diligently with a CBT therapist for several months, and you've made incredible strides in managing your anxiety, challenging negative thought patterns, and building healthier relationships. You feel more confident, empowered, and in control of your life than ever before. But as your therapy sessions come to an end, you start to worry. Will you be able to maintain this progress on your own? What if you slip back into old habits and patterns of thinking? These concerns are common and understandable, but it's important to remember that with the right strategies and mindset, you can absolutely maintain your progress and continue to grow and thrive.

Maintaining progress is crucial because it helps you to solidify the positive changes you've made and integrate them into your daily life. When you consistently practice and reinforce the CBT techniques you've learned, they become more automatic and habitual, making it easier to maintain your progress over time. This is similar to learning any new skill, like playing an instrument or speaking a foreign language. The more you practice, the more natural and effortless it becomes.

Preventing relapse is equally important, as it helps you to avoid slipping back into old, unhelpful patterns of thinking and behavior that can undermine your progress and well-being. Relapse is a common experience in the journey of personal growth and change, and it's important to remember that it's not a sign of failure. Rather, it's an opportunity to learn, adjust, and strengthen your skills and resilience. By being proactive and prepared for the possibility of relapse, you can minimize its impact and get back on track more quickly.

The Challenges of Maintaining Progress and Preventing Relapse

Maintaining progress and preventing relapse can be challenging for a variety of reasons. Here are some of the common obstacles that women may face:

1 Life stressors and transitions: As women, we often juggle multiple roles and responsibilities, such as work, family, and caregiving. Life can be unpredictable, and stressors such as job changes, relationship difficulties, or health issues can arise unexpectedly. These

challenges can make it harder to prioritize self-care and maintain the gains made through CBT.

Example: Julia, a 35-year-old mother of two, had been making great progress in managing her anxiety and setting healthy boundaries in her relationships. However, when her mother was diagnosed with a serious illness and required additional care, Julia found herself feeling overwhelmed and struggling to maintain her own self-care practices. She began to slip back into old patterns of people-pleasing and neglecting her own needs.

2 Negative self-talk and self-doubt: Even after making significant progress through CBT, negative self-talk and self-doubt can still creep in. It's easy to fall back into old habits of self-criticism or to question whether the changes you've made are truly sustainable.

Example: Samantha, a 28-year-old entrepreneur, had worked hard to challenge her perfectionism and build a more balanced and fulfilling life. However, when she encountered a setback in her business, she found herself falling back into negative self-talk and questioning her abilities. She began to doubt whether she had really made any lasting changes.

3 Lack of support or accountability: Maintaining progress can be more difficult when you don't have a strong support system or sense of accountability. Without regular check-ins or encouragement from others, it can be easy to lose motivation or let old habits resurface.

Example: Priya, a 42-year-old teacher, had made significant strides in assertiveness and boundary setting through her CBT work. However, when her therapy sessions ended, she found it challenging to maintain her progress on her own. She missed the regular support and accountability of meeting with her therapist and began to slip back into old patterns of avoidance and passivity.

4 Complacency or overconfidence: Sometimes, when we've made significant progress, it's easy to become complacent or overconfident. We may think that we've "arrived" and no longer need to be as proactive or vigilant in maintaining our gains.

Example: Mei, a 50-year-old executive, had worked hard to overcome her impostor syndrome and build greater self-confidence in her leadership abilities. After receiving a major promotion, she began to feel like she had finally "made it" and no longer needed to prioritize her personal growth and self-care. She became less proactive in practicing the CBT techniques that had helped her get to this point.

While these challenges are common, they are not insurmountable. With the right strategies and mindset, you can navigate these obstacles and continue to thrive in your personal growth and empowerment journey. Let's explore some practical, long-term CBT strategies for maintaining progress and preventing relapse.

Long-Term CBT Strategies for Maintaining Progress and Preventing Relapse

1 Develop a maintenance plan: One of the most effective ways to maintain your progress is to develop a personalized maintenance plan. This plan should include the specific CBT techniques and strategies that have been most helpful for you, as well as a schedule for practicing and reinforcing these skills. Your maintenance plan might include:

• Regular self-reflection and journaling to monitor your thoughts, emotions, and behaviors

• Scheduled "check-ins" with yourself to assess your progress and identify areas for continued growth

• Ongoing practice of techniques such as cognitive restructuring, behavioral activation, and relaxation strategies

• A list of healthy coping mechanisms and self-care practices to turn to in times of stress

Example: After completing her CBT treatment for social anxiety, Lila worked with her therapist to develop a maintenance plan. Her plan included daily thought records to monitor and challenge anxious thoughts, weekly exposure practices to continue building confidence in social situations, and regular self-care activities like meditation and exercise. By having a concrete plan in place, Lila felt more prepared and empowered to maintain her progress.

2 Stay engaged in meaningful activities: Engaging in activities that bring a sense of purpose, mastery, and enjoyment can help you to maintain your progress and prevent relapse. When we're actively

engaged in pursuits that matter to us, we're less likely to fall back into old, unhelpful patterns of thinking and behavior.

Example: Through her CBT work, Nadia had rediscovered her love of painting and found that it was a powerful tool for managing her depression. As part of her long-term maintenance plan, Nadia committed to setting aside time each week to work on her art, either alone or in a class or group. She found that staying engaged in this meaningful activity not only brought her joy and fulfillment, but also helped her to maintain her progress in managing her mental health.

3 Build and maintain a support system: Having a strong support system is crucial for maintaining progress and preventing relapse. Surround yourself with people who understand and support your personal growth journey, and who can offer encouragement, accountability, and a listening ear when needed.

Example: Jasmine had always struggled with opening up to others about her mental health, but through her CBT work, she had learned the importance of vulnerability and connection. As part of her long-term maintenance plan, Jasmine joined a women's support group where she could continue to practice sharing her experiences and receiving support. She also made a commitment to regularly check in with a few trusted friends and family members about her progress and any challenges she was facing.

4 Practice self-compassion and acceptance: Self-compassion and acceptance are key ingredients for maintaining progress and preventing relapse. When we approach ourselves with kindness, understanding, and acceptance, we're better able to navigate challenges and setbacks without falling into self-blame or giving up altogether.

Example: Raina had made significant progress in overcoming her perfectionism and building self-esteem through CBT. However, she still found herself getting caught up in self-criticism when she made mistakes or fell short of her own high expectations. As part of her long-term maintenance plan, Raina committed to practicing self-compassion by treating herself with the same kindness and understanding she would offer a good friend. She also worked on accepting that setbacks and imperfections were a normal part of the growth process, rather than signs of failure.

5 Continue learning and growing: Maintaining progress and preventing relapse is an ongoing process, and there is always room for continued learning and growth. Stay curious and open to new ideas, insights, and strategies that can support your personal growth journey.

Example: After completing her initial CBT work, Elena made a commitment to continue learning about personal growth and mental health. She read books and articles on topics like mindfulness, resilience, and healthy relationships, and attended workshops and seminars when possible. By staying engaged in ongoing learning, Elena found that she was able to continually deepen her self-awareness and expand her toolkit of strategies for maintaining her well-being.

6 Celebrate your progress and successes: Celebrating your progress and successes, no matter how small, is a powerful way to maintain momentum and motivation in your personal growth journey. Take time to acknowledge and appreciate the positive changes you've made and the challenges you've overcome.

Example: Sasha had a tendency to downplay her accomplishments and focus on what she still needed to improve. Through her CBT work, she had learned to challenge this negative bias and cultivate a more balanced and appreciative perspective. As part of her long-term maintenance plan, Sasha started a "success journal" where she recorded her daily wins and progress, no matter how small. She also made a point of sharing her successes with her support system and celebrating milestones along the way.

7 Be proactive in managing stress and triggers: Being proactive in managing stress and triggers is key to maintaining progress and preventing relapse. Identify your personal triggers and early warning signs of stress or setbacks, and develop a plan for coping with these challenges in healthy ways.

Example: Tanya had a history of turning to alcohol and overeating when stressed or overwhelmed. Through her CBT work, she had developed healthier coping mechanisms and learned to identify her triggers. As part of her long-term maintenance plan, Tanya made a list of her top stress triggers, such as work deadlines or family conflicts, and developed a specific plan for managing each one. This included strategies like breaking tasks into smaller steps, practicing assertive communication, and using relaxation techniques like deep breathing or progressive muscle relaxation.

8 Be willing to seek additional support when needed: Maintaining progress and preventing relapse doesn't mean you have to do it all on your own. Be willing to seek additional support from a therapist, support group, or other resources if you find yourself struggling or in need of extra guidance.

Example: Carla had made great strides in managing her anxiety and building healthier relationships through CBT. However, when she went through a difficult divorce, she found herself struggling to cope and slipping back into old patterns of negative thinking and avoidance. Rather than trying to tough it out on her own, Carla reached out to her former CBT therapist for a few "booster" sessions to help her navigate this challenging time and reinforce her coping skills.

Remember, seeking additional support is a sign of strength and self-awareness, not weakness. It takes courage and wisdom to know when you need extra help and to reach out for it.

Conclusion and Final Thoughts

Maintaining progress and preventing relapse is an ongoing process that requires commitment, self-awareness, and a proactive approach. By developing a personalized maintenance plan, staying engaged in meaningful activities, building a strong support system, practicing self-compassion, continuing to learn and grow, celebrating your successes, being proactive in managing stress and triggers, and being willing to seek additional support when needed, you can sustain the positive changes you've made through CBT and continue to thrive in your personal growth journey.

Remember, setbacks and challenges are a normal part of the growth process. When you encounter obstacles or slip back into old patterns, don't beat yourself up or give up. Instead, treat these moments as opportunities for learning, self-reflection, and recommitment to your goals and values.

Celebrate how far you've come and trust in your own resilience and capacity for change. You have the tools, the strengths, and the wisdom within you to navigate life's challenges and to create a life that is authentic, fulfilling, and true to who you are.

As you continue on your personal growth and empowerment journey, remember to be patient, compassionate, and kind with yourself. Embrace the ups and downs, the victories and the setbacks, as all part of the beautiful, messy, and rewarding process of growth and self-discovery.

And know that you are not alone. There is a community of women out there who are walking this path alongside you, cheering you on, and ready to support you every step of the way. Reach out, connect, and lean on each other as you continue to learn, grow, and thrive.

You've got this. You are capable of incredible things. Keep going, keep growing, and never stop believing in yourself and your ability to create a life of meaning, purpose, and joyful empowerment. The world needs your unique gifts, your authentic voice, and your courageous heart. Shine on, sister. Your journey is just beginning.